the balance plan

Six Steps to Optimize Your Hormonal Health

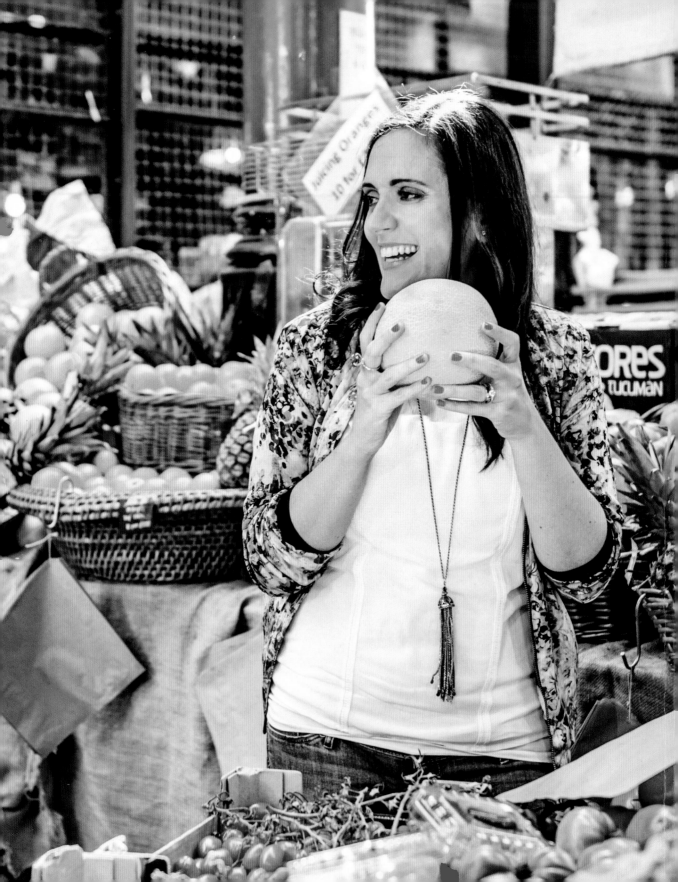

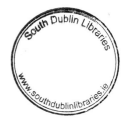

the balance plan

Six Steps to Optimize Your Hormonal Health

Angelique Panagos

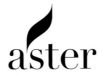

aster

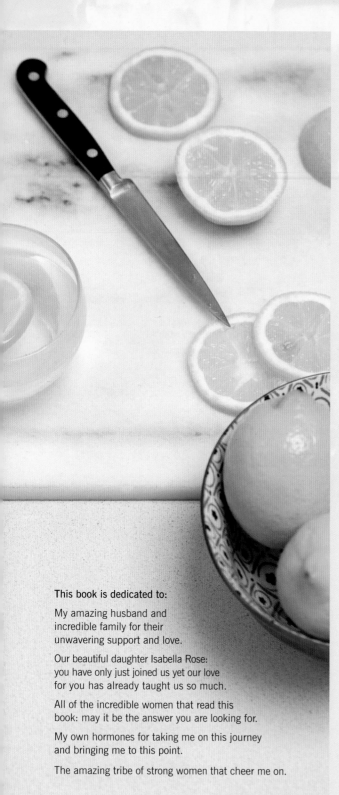

An Hachette UK Company
www.hachette.co.uk

First published in Great Britain in 2017 by Aster,
an imprint of Octopus Publishing Group Ltd
Carmelite House, 50 Victoria Embankment
London EC4Y 0DZ
www.octopusbooks.co.uk

This edition published in 2018

ISBN 978-1-91202-378-3

A CIP catalogue record for this book is available from the
British Library.

Printed and bound in China

10 9 8 7 6 5 4 3 2 1

Publishing Director: Stephanie Jackson
Contributing Editor: Hannah Ebelthite
Editor: Pollyanna Poulter
Art Director: Juliette Norsworthy
Designer: Lizzie Ballantyne
Photographers: Clare Winfield and Ian Sidebottom
Prop Stylist: Jennifer Kay
Home Economist and Food Stylist: Emily Kydd
Production Manager: Caroline Alberti

Disclaimer

All reasonable care has been taken in the preparation of this
book, but the information it contains is not intended to take the
place of treatment by a qualified medical practitioner. Before
making any changes in your health regime, always consult
a doctor. You must seek professional advice if you are in any
doubt about any medical condition. Any application of the ideas
and information contained in this book is at the reader's sole
discretion and risk. Neither Octopus Publishing Group Limited or
the author take any responsibility for any consequences resulting
from the use or misuse of information contained in this book.

This book is dedicated to:

My amazing husband and
incredible family for their
unwavering support and love.

Our beautiful daughter Isabella Rose:
you have only just joined us yet our love
for you has already taught us so much.

All of the incredible women that read this
book: may it be the answer you are looking for.

My own hormones for taking me on this journey
and bringing me to this point.

The amazing tribe of strong women that cheer me on.

Contents

Introduction

My journey into nutrition and hormonal health hasn't been one of being super-healthy my whole life with perfectly balanced hormones. No, on the contrary, it has been one of self-sabotage, healing and discovery. Monthly cycles can be a crazy roller-coaster ride you feel you cannot escape, and my introduction to hormones at the age of ten (my first menstrual period) was no exception.

It was a troubled relationship from the outset – I was the girl who went home from school, and later from work, with period pains and debilitating headaches. The girl whose moods were mercurial and whose bloating was out of control. I suffered insomnia, turning to caffeine, sugar and diet soda to keep myself awake. My weight and self-esteem fluctuated from one month to the next; I felt like I had to tuck my top and my stomach into my trousers! I was totally disconnected from my body. We were strangers, enemies even. As my weight ballooned, I would numb my toxic moods and extreme fatigue with alcohol, junk food and sugar. My periods became so sporadic, I couldn't identify a proper menstrual cycle any more.

In my early twenties, at my heaviest weight (and lowest mood), I was determined to take radical control of my body. I exercised obsessively and curbed my eating, which led to anorexia and bulimia. My periods stopped for six months and my hair even started falling out. I developed Hashimoto's, an autoimmune hypothyroidism, a condition in which my thyroid attacked itself. When I started eating again, I couldn't stop. No matter how hard I tried, the cravings won and my weight skyrocketed, though I continued exercising obsessively.

For most of my twenties, I was bloated, exhausted and continuously premenstrual, although I didn't have periods for three months at a time. I was 20 kilos overweight and was diagnosed with polycystic ovary syndrome (PCOS). I felt alone, exhausted and desperate. I finally took control at the age of twenty-seven, taking small, consistent steps to change my beliefs around food, and to educate myself about nutrition and hormonal balance. I learned not only how stress and poor nutrition wreak havoc on our hormones, but also how vital gut health and proper digestion are to our overall wellbeing. I lost 18 kilos and started menstruating regularly – a massive improvement in mind and body.

My greatest learning has been that working to optimize my hormones is a journey, a series of gentle, consistent changes over time. This is my message: a lifestyle that achieves hormonal balance is about consistency, not perfection. It's about nourishment, not deprivation. Now I honour my body by respecting its natural cycle, working with it instead of against it.

This healing journey is not over. I struggled to get pregnant and, like so many, have experienced miscarriage, unfortunately two of them, before being blessed with our beautiful daughter. But this further deepens my passion to help women understand and support their hormonal balance. I consider hormonal balance more of a lifestyle evolution: small, considered steps over time. We do not need to dread and numb our cycles; we can create balance-sustaining hormonal health over our lifetimes. We can educate ourselves, support each other, learn to celebrate our feminine cycle and feel better and more vibrant than ever. It's never too late.

My story, if anything, attests to the body's amazing resilience when we honour our hormonal health.

Angelique
x

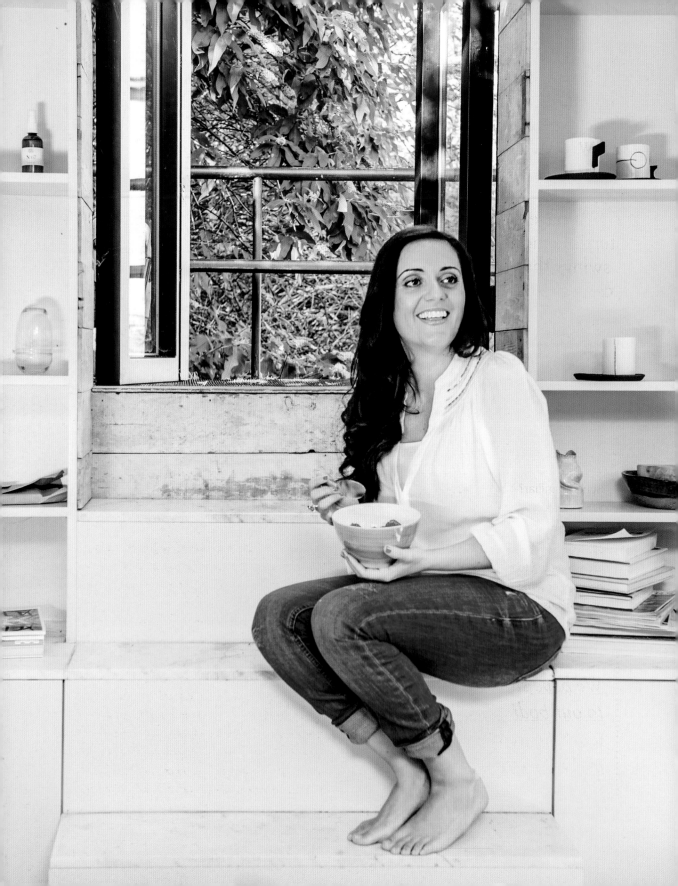

How do You Feel?

'I feel exhausted'

'I need my daily fix of chocolate'

'I have terrible mood swings that I can't control'

'I'm hungrier than I used to be, but never feel satisfied when I eat more'

'Sex drive? What sex drive?'

'I struggle to lose weight no matter what I try'

Sound familiar? You are not alone. These are complaints that I hear every day. Time and time again, they're caused by the same thing – hormonal imbalance.

Many of the women who come to my clinic are struggling to feel good, and are puzzled because nothing seems to work. Almost none of them suspects that a hormonal imbalance might be the cause of their anguish. Instead, these women question their willpower, blame themselves and feel frustrated that this is their 'normal'.

We have stopped listening to our bodies and working with their natural, cyclical rhythms

Let's face it: we are stressed, exhausted and feel a low-grade variety of awful pretty consistently, especially during our menstrual cycle. This general malaise is not severe enough for us to see a doctor, necessarily, but it can make life less fulfilling than it could be. When we feel stressed and fatigued for so long, we forget how good we can actually feel. We have stopped listening to our bodies and working with their natural, cyclical rhythms, and instead

Symptoms You Might Recognize

Surprisingly, hormonal imbalances might appear as:

— insomnia
— constipation
— flatulence
— skin breakouts
— acne
— exhaustion
— thinning hair
— weight gain
— anxiety
— headaches
— migraines
— PMS
— heavy, painful or irrregular periods
— low (or no) sex drive
— forgetfulness
— depression
— tearfulness
— irritability
— poor tolerance to stress
— low mood
— mood swings
— food cravings
— oily hair
— brain fog
— tender breasts
— lumpy breasts
— lack of motivation
— cold hands and feet
— bloating and loose stools

we numb or stimulate ourselves with sugar, refined foods and caffeine. We have become disconnected from our bodies. The price we pay for this disconnection and fast living is feeling low-energy, lethargic and out of balance most, if not all, of the time.

The problem is made worse when we consume foods that are high in convenience but low in nutrients. Add to this that we are sleeping less and stressing more, often without any consistent relaxation. Our delicate hormonal balance is disrupted when we are constantly 'on'.

Hormones seem mysterious things, filling many women with dread around 'that time of the month'. Periods have become notorious times of rampant mood swings and insatiable cravings, times when many women feel they are not their usual selves. So many women just succumb to feeling this way because they don't know how to change it longer-term. Their strategy is to fight it, short-term, with pain killers, sugar or caffeine. Part of the problem is that most of us know almost nothing about how our hormones work, so we don't work with them. Our hormones affect everything from our menstrual cycle (and all the challenges that may come with it, like heavy bleeding, cravings and irritability) to health issues including fibroids, miscarriages, infertility, polycystic ovary syndrome (PCOS) and endometriosis.

How the Balance Plan Can Help

The aim of this book is to invite you to be part of a new conversation that we are having about hormones, to look at it from a different angle – addressing the underlying cause, creating balance and not just covering it with a plaster and hoping it goes away. I will help you understand why you are feeling exhausted, irritable and overweight, and I'll tell you what you can do about it. Together, we will bring balance and vibrancy back into your life, and reclaim your body.

I will take you through my six-step method for creating optimal hormonal balance. You will learn about the medicinal power of food, with delicious new recipes to try in my 28-day programme. You will also learn lifestyle tweaks – small, consistent changes done over time that will 'evolution-ize' your hormonal health. This is not a fad diet or a quick fix. It's not about rigid rules or perfection. This is a sustainable, long-term solution that has worked for me, and for many others.

Whatever your motivation, when your hormones are in check you'll be more excited about yourself, your life and your possibilities

I want to support you too! Whatever your motivation, when your hormones are in check you'll be more excited about yourself, your life and your possibilities. Whether you are looking to feel more balanced and energized throughout the month, have a healthy pregnancy, get through menopause relatively symptom-free, or simply optimize your hormonal health at any age, this book is for you.

Ready to Transform Your Life?

Get ready to tune in to your hormones and make the changes necessary to bring them into balance. Take the six steps, follow the 28-day plan, transform your life and:

— sleep better
— reduce stress
— enhance digestion
— elevate energy levels
— lose weight
— feel happier

Welcome to the Hormone Balance Plan

Finally stepping off my own hormone roller-coaster in my late 20s is what led me to create the Hormone Balance Plan. I wanted to help other people realize what complex beings us women are, and how easily our hormonal balance can be disrupted – but also how easily the right diet and lifestyle choice can make a positive difference. I tested the plan out on myself and my family first, and saw such profound results that I had to share the method with everyone who needed it. I couldn't keep it to myself, and my clinic was a good place to start. My goal as a nutritionist was to get people to a place where they didn't need me any longer, where they had seen the results and learnt the tools to unleash their healing potential and continue to live this new lifestyle of hormonal evolution as they easily glided through the different phases of life.

The method, which is grounded in nutrition and functional medicine, has shown phenomenal results in women with irregular, painful and heavy periods, headaches, low libido, bone loss, ovarian cysts, fibroids, mood issues, insomnia, stubborn weight gain, extreme fatigue, the dreaded PMS, cystitis, endometriosis, PCOS, fertility concerns and, in postpartum, perimenopausal or menopausal women. As it's flexible, I can adapt it to the unique biochemical individuality of each woman.

Now I can share it with you all. Together we will create a healthy tribe of supportive women who are free of hormonal turmoil, and I am honoured to be here with you.

The Plan – an Overview

In this book, we will explore how your hormones work, focussing on those that I call the Sassy Six (*see* Part 1; pages 14–31). We will also expose seven Showstoppers (*see* Part 2; pages 32–55) – the most common disruptors of hormonal balance. The key to the Balance Plan, and what we will delve into next, consists of the following Six Pillars of hormonal balance (explored in more detail in Part 3, *see* pages 56–81):

Pillar One: Nourish
For optimal function, hormones need to be provided with a constant supply of nutrients from the food we eat. Unfortunately our current Western diet falls short in a big way! My aim is to change the way we think about food. Consistent achievable changes to our diet can make a huge difference to our hormonal balance, virtually straight away. What we eat really is that powerful.

Pillar Two: Balance
Creating and maintaining blood-sugar balance helps to stabilize our hormones. This leads

to better moods, easier sleep, reduced PMS and less tummy fat. This Pillar is also about balancing the digestive system. About 80 per cent of the women who come to see me have a digestive issue, or discomfort. There is a strong correlation between gut health and hormonal health.

Pillar Three: Nurture

The message of stress overrides any other message in the body. Too much or too little cortisol, the stress hormone, unbalances our hormones. For example, it affects thyroid function, which can lead to fatigue, weight gain and hair loss. So this Pillar is about giving our stress and master metabolism glands (the adrenal and thyroid glands) some TLC.

Pillar Four: Cleanse

Extensive research has shown many links between environmental toxins and our hormones, especially as the liver is responsible for the packaging and removal of spent hormones. Pillar Four is about cleansing the body – and our environment – of its toxic burden.

Pillar Five: Move

Exercise is essential for hormonal health. We lead more sedentary lifestyles with convenience at an all-time high and it's having an adverse effect on our hormones and health; so much so that sitting is deemed to be 'the new smoking'. It is the quality and amount of movement that are important. This Pillar helps you find that sweet spot.

Pillar Six: Restore

This is all about creating the inner peace that is so important for stress reduction, improved mood and good digestion, all of which contribute to hormonal balance. We work on getting better sleep, for repair and healing, as well as 'me time', meditation and gratitude.

Once I've taken you through the Six Pillars and how to create and maintain them, we'll look at the nutrition foundations that underpin my plan. In Part 4 (*see* pages 82–105), we take measurements, make sure you're fully prepared and start a food diary. I'll give you all the knowledge you need to follow my four-week menu, along with advice on what to eat when you're out and about – and, crucially, how to continue once the four weeks are over.

I absolutely love my work and the privilege of meeting so many inspiring women, and I am excited to accompany you on this journey, to meet and live in harmony with your hormones. So, let's get started…

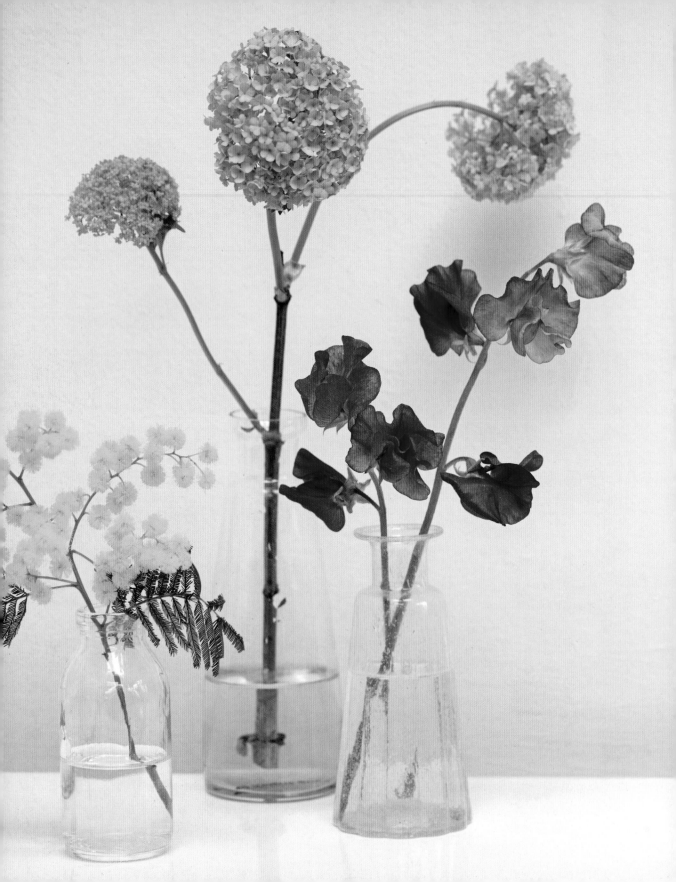

how hormones work

Hormones 101

If your menstrual cycle is the dance, then where does the music come from? Consider your hormones like a symphony, conducted by the endocrine system, which is made up of a number of glands and organs. These include the hypothalamus, pituitary gland, thyroid, pancreas, adrenal glands and ovaries (in females), and the testes (in males). They may seem unrelated, but they communicate and work together, the way different instruments make up an orchestra.

Your glands control important physiological functions by releasing powerful chemical messengers (hormones) into the blood. The word 'hormone' comes from a Greek word *hormon*, meaning 'set in motion', and that's precisely what your hormones do: they trigger activity in different organs and body parts.

A Delicate Balance

It's an intricate three-tier system that works like an efficiently run company – the hypothalamus in the brain is the MD and will release a stimulating or inhibitory hormone message to the pituitary (the manager), telling it what needs to be done, and the pituitary then communicates through hormone messages with the other endocrine organs (the workforce), and instructs them what to do. Once this chain reaction is complete, there is what's called a feedback loop, where the end organ hormones feed back to the hypothalamus. This message

is just as important, as it reports back the current hormone levels so that the hypothalamus can give the next command – and so the cycle continues.

Meet the Sassy Six

Now there are many hormones at work in your body, but there are six key players that I want you to be familiar with. I call them the Sassy Six, because they each play key roles in making you feel like your sassy self. They are: progesterone, testosterone, oestrogen, cortisol, thyroid and insulin. No hormone works in isolation; they work in synergy and, ideally, in balance.

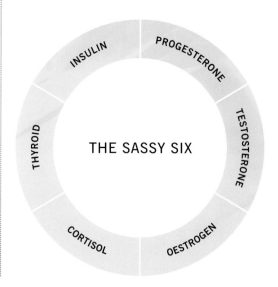

INSULIN PROGESTERONE TESTOSTERONE OESTROGEN CORTISOL THYROID

THE SASSY SIX

The first four of our Sassy Six are classified as steroid (or steroidal) hormones. Steroid hormones are derived from lipids, specifically fats, cholesterol and circulating LDL (what's referred to as 'bad' cholesterol) in the bloodstream. In the liver, this cholesterol is used to make a precursor steroid hormone called pregnenolone. From pregnenolone we synthesize our other steroid hormones. So it's important for hormone production that we have the right fats in our diet and that our liver is functioning optimally. Converting cholesterol to pregnenolone is an energy-intensive process, and cellular energy comes from a nutrient-dense diet. Thyroid and insulin are peptide hormones and are synthesized from proteins (amino acids) with the help of nutrients known as co-factors, such as B vitamins or selenium. Already you can see the importance of food when it comes to hormone health.

No Fat? No Thanks

Forget low-fat or no-fat diets. Why? Because your sex hormones are made from lipids, aka fats. If you don't get enough essential fats from the food you eat, your body cannot make adequate levels of oestrogen, progesterone and testosterone. These sex hormones are essential to life and to feeling confident, vibrant and energetic.

So what happens if your hormones are not in balance? All sorts of symptoms can result, but here are just a few examples:

— low progesterone can lead to irregular menstrual cycles, irritability, infertility, miscarriage, insomnia and PMS
— low testosterone can lead to low self-esteem, weight gain, low libido and moodiness
— high testosterone can lead to irritability, weight gain, infertility, anger, facial hair and acne
— low oestrogen can lead to headaches, panic attacks, low mood and libido, bone loss, vaginal dryness and belly fat
— high oestrogen can cause breast tenderness, PMS, heavy periods, fibroids, endometriosis, cysts and even breast cancer
— low cortisol makes you feel burnt-out, exhausted and drained, tearful, PMS, taking you from superhero to super cranky
— high cortisol causes that tired, but wired feeling, anxiety, insomnia and belly fat
— low thyroid can cause brain fog, fatigue, weight gain, constipation, cold hands and feet, thinning hair and miscarriage
— elevated insulin can lead to that dreaded muffin top, PMS, constant hunger, excess testosterone, elevated cortisol, insulin resistance and Type 2 diabetes

Before we explore each of the Sassy Six, their roles and what can happen if they're not in balance, let's take a look at the monthly hormonal dance that is the female cycle…

Our Monthly Hormonal Dance

When balanced, our hormones can create a beautiful, synchronized dance, like a graceful Viennese waltz. But for many of us, that monthly dance is more like doing the hokey cokey, using the wrong feet! The purpose of this dance is for our body to prepare itself for a possible pregnancy each and every cycle. This is pretty incredible; it's the true essence of our feminine power and I believe it should be embraced. By understanding our cycle and helping to bring it into balance, the dance becomes more graceful. Menstruation (the bleed) is just one part of the cycle, which runs for anything from 21 to 35 days (although I would like to see you closer to 25 to 35 days). Let's take a look at each of the three phases.

1. The Follicular Phase

I like to divide the follicular phase (also known as the proliferation phase) into two parts: menstruation and the pre-ovulatory phase. It all starts with menstruation, from the first day of our bleed as we start to shed the previous month's lining (if there's no pregnancy), and this part lasts anything from three to seven days.

Hormone Activity

Our main menstruation hormones are low at this point. The brain's hypothalamus releases gonadotropin-releasing hormone (GnRH), which tells the pituitary gland to produce follicle-stimulating hormone (FSH), and this is the start of the pre-ovulatory phase, which lasts seven to ten days. FSH hormone races through the blood to reach the ovaries, and once there it stimulates the development of the eggs in the follicles of the ovaries. Each follicle contains a single egg, and each month several follicles start to develop their eggs, but only one egg will reign supreme. The maturing follicles have also started producing oestrogen, which stimulates the thickening of the womb lining (the endometrium) in preparation for the possible implantation of a fertilized egg.

Noticeable Changes

You may notice a feeling of relief as menstruation begins, possibly followed by restlessness or irritability, especially if you experience a lot of cramps, and a slight dip in your energy. You may notice a surge in energy around days two and three, when oestrogen starts to increase again. Nearing the end of this phase, your cervical fluid (discharge) will take on a wetter, more milky consistency that looks and feels creamy.

2. The Ovulatory Phase

This is the big event of the cycle – what it has all been leading up to! For many, this part of the cycle starts in the second week and is the shortest phase, lasting only two to four days. As our follicles produce more oestrogen, further thickening and preparing the womb lining, it reaches a peak which is detected by the pituitary gland. In response, the pituitary gland releases a burst of luteinizing hormone (LH), known as an 'LH surge'. This surge is the trigger for the dominant egg to fully mature and be released from the follicle, to be swept away into a fallopian tube where it will survive for 12 to 24 hours. If fertilization doesn't occur, the egg is reabsorbed by the body or excreted with our next menstrual flow.

Hormone Activity

There is a sharp rise in testosterone as we head for ovulation, but this is short-lived. If fertilization occurs, we start producing human chorionic gonadotropin (hCG), which is the hormone most pregnancy tests detect. The hCG hormone initially produced by the embryo signals to the corpus luteum to keep making progesterone and oestrogen in order to maintain the pregnancy.

Noticeable Changes

Energy levels are distinctly higher, and the rise in testosterone enhances sex drive and zest for life – you may feel more confident and find yourself initiating sex more. Cervical fluid will feel wetter – it's clear at this point, with the texture of raw egg white, and can be pulled between the fingers. This signals that ovulation is pending, and you may notice a slight bloody discharge, which is referred to as ovulatory spotting. You may feel a dull or sharp pain in your lower abdomen, known as ovulatory pain. Your temperature increases slightly with ovulation.

3. The Luteal Phase

The luteal phase (or the post-ovulatory or secretory phase) is the longest and usually lasts 12 to 14 days. The dominant follicle from which the egg bursts has another important function and collapses to become a transient endocrine gland, the corpus luteum (meaning 'yellow body'). It remains on the wall of the ovary.

Hormone Activity

The corpus luteum starts to produce progesterone. Progesterone prevents the release of another egg for the rest of that cycle, signalling to the pituitary to stop producing FSH and LH so that only one egg is released; it also causes the endometrium to thicken and to fill with fluids and nutrients in order to nourish a potential embryo. Levels of progesterone and oestrogen are still high at this stage (progesterone is about 200 times higher), and testosterone will surge again shortly, but if the egg is not fertilized the corpus luteum will collapse and be reabsorbed. At this stage, there is a drop in both oestrogen and progesterone, and we start to shed our lining, taking us to the start of a new cycle.

Noticeable Changes

Progesterone causes our body temperature to remain slightly elevated. Cervical mucus becomes stickier, drier and cloudy. In the second half of this phase you may notice a drop in energy, due to the calming effects of progesterone. Unfortunately, this phase often also comes with PMS symptoms such as bloating, sore breasts, insomnia and cravings.

Progesterone

– the Zen master

Derived from our mother hormone, pregnenolone, progesterone helps prepare our body for conception and pregnancy, while regulating the menstrual cycle. It is produced in large amounts in the ovaries during the luteal phase of our monthly waltz, in the placenta if we are pregnant, and in the adrenal glands in small amounts throughout life.

Progesterone has positive effects on:
— building bones
— balancing oestrogen (another of the Sassy Six)
— breast health
— cardiovascular health
— nervous system health
— brain function
— preventing anxiety, irritability, PMS and mood swings
— sleep
— the GABA receptors in our brain

It's also a precursor hormone: there are receptor sites for progesterone throughout our body, waiting for it to come floating by, and three of our other Sassy Six can be made from it – testosterone, oestrogen and cortisol.

Causes of Imbalance

The body is constantly deciding whether to make more sex hormones like progesterone, testosterone and oestrogen, or more stress hormones like cortisol. We are genetically programmed to allow stress to override any other message in the body, because it might signal an acute life or death situation. Yet we are not living the life that we are genetically programmed to live. Instead, we are living in a state of chronic stress, which equates to a signal of 'SOS, skip progesterone to make the cortisol, I need to live, this woman is constantly under attack!' This action is often referred to as the 'pregnenolone steal' (or the progesterone or cortisol steal): in very basic terms, if a woman is stressed, whether emotionally or physically, her body favours the production of cortisol, which can lead to sub-optimal pregnenolone and progesterone levels and in turn not enough raw material to make the other sex hormones.

Although stress is a major player, it is not the only cause of our progesterone level being sub-optimal. Others include:
— genetic factors
— luteal phase defect
— ageing

- perimenopause
- menopause
- low thyroid (another of our Sassy Six)
- PCOS
- deficiencies in vitamins and minerals such as magnesium, vitamins A, B6 and C, and zinc
- high prolactin
- low LH hormone
- eating disorders
- a nutrient-poor diet
- high sugar consumption (that's right, biscuits, I am looking at you!)

Results of Progesterone Imbalance

- imbalances in the monthly cycle
- heavy flow during menstruation
- spotting between periods
- miscarriage
- osteoporosis
- PMS
- mood swings/irritability
- anxiety
- insomnia

When we produce the right amount of progesterone we function better, our cycle is easier and we feel more even-tempered, relaxed, and calm

Remedies

It's important to evaluate and see what lifestyle changes we can make to bring progesterone back into balance. Taking a pill or slathering on cream (as in oral contraceptives, hormone replacement therapy, or HRT) is not the first step. That's the replacement model, but we want to approach things from the functional model – making lasting lifestyle changes to correct the underlying causes of the imbalance. The Six Pillars of Balance, on pages 60–81, are your starting point.

Progesterone and Osteoporosis

Progesterone (and oestrogen) deficiency can seriously affect bone health and is of great concern in the development of osteoporosis. When I was at the height of the anorexia, I stopped menstruating for over six months – a condition referred to as amenorrhea. When I discussed this with a doctor, he explained that because my body weight was so low, I did not have the raw materials to make the hormones and nutrients needed to support my bone health. This was causing a decrease in new bone formation (osteoblast activity), and without sorting this out I was on a slippery path to brittle and fragile bones.

Testosterone

– the king of va-va-voom

Most women I speak to don't even think of testosterone as being part of the female hormonal soup. Let's blow the lid on that one – yes, testosterone is commonly referred to as a 'male hormone', but it falls into a class of hormones called androgens, and women have androgens, too. When in balance, these androgens have a positive effect on:

— vigour
— mood
— memory
— strengthening ligaments
— building muscle and bone
— brain function
— assertive behaviour
— sense of wellbeing
— self-confidence
— libido

Calling testosterone a 'male hormone' is a misnomer – sorry, boys, you don't have the monopoly

Testosterone is made in the adrenal glands and ovaries (although at a much lower level than is made in the testes and adrenals in men), and has an important role in our menstrual cycle. Testosterone is converted into oestrogen, making it extremely important for female hormone balance. This happens via an enzyme called aromatase, which is found in many tissues, such as the adrenal glands, ovaries, placenta, adipose (fat) tissue and brain.

Testosterone is kept in check by a clever protein made in the liver called sex hormone binding globulin (SHBG), which binds up free testosterone so that it doesn't charge around the bloodstream and cause havoc.

Causes of Imbalance

Too Much Testosterone

High insulin causes the ovaries to create more testosterone, to speed up aromatase activity and to decrease SHBG. And high insulin levels are caused by an over-consumption of sugary, refined foods and stimulants. So we get more free testosterone whizzing around the body and more oestrogen being made, which can also lead to weight gain and excess oestrogen/oestrogen dominance.

The more fat cells you have, the more aromatase is stimulated and the greater the decrease in SHBG – and so the vicious cycle continues.

Over-exercising is another cause of elevated androgens and testosterone, as is a poor diet high in refined carbohydrates, sugar and low in fats, vegetables and protein.

Too Little Testosterone

Stress diverts pregnenolone into that cortisol pathway, and it takes away the raw material to make androgens and testosterone.

Other factors that can lower testosterone levels in women include low-fat diets, depression, endometriosis, menopause, environmental toxins, lack of exercise and psychological trauma.

The Pill and Low Libido

The contraceptive pill increases SHBG, and even though this might sound like a positive, elevated SHBG will bind too much free testosterone, making it inactive. Therefore, when SHBG goes up in the body, it lowers the amount of free testosterone – not good for your libido and energy. We need an optimal amount of SHBG so that we don't have either too much or too little free testosterone. I know, I know, it's complicated.

Results of Testosterone Imbalance

— oily skin
— acne
— excess hair on the face and body (hirsutism)
— fatigue
— sagging skin
— anxiety
— depression
— weight gain
— male pattern baldness
— menstrual irregularity
— low sex drive
— fertility issues
— in some cases PCOS

Remedies

Think about your current lifestyle, diet and how you react to stress, all of which are addressed in our Six Pillars – <u>Pillar One: Nourish, Pillar Two: Balance and Pillar Three: Nurture (*see* pages 60–71) will be key for you.</u>

Oestrogen
– the awkward triplets

Oestrogen is a collective name for a group of hormones, and the three major naturally occurring oestrogens in women are oestrone (E1), oestradiol (E2) and oestriol (E3) – hence the 'triplets'. But we'll keep it simple and refer to them all as oestrogen. Produced mainly in the ovaries but also by the adrenal glands and in the fat tissues, and by the placenta during pregnancy, oestrogen is the hormone that makes us female. It not only ensures our menstruation cycle runs smoothly, it bestows on us breasts, hips, soft skin, pubic hair, the maturation of the skeleton and even influences the feminine pitch of our voices.

We have oestrogen receptors everywhere in our body: in our brain, bones, gut, breasts, heart, lungs, bladder, muscles, ovaries and vagina. These receptors are essential for oestrogen to perform over 300 functions in the body. As well as those already mentioned, they include:

Feeling fat around the middle? Excess oestrogen could be a cause

— maintaining bone density and muscle mass
— protecting the brain
— having a positive effect on our mood by aiding the formation of serotonin
— keeping skin supple and young-looking by maintaining collagen and water content
— protecting our heart by keeping our arteries open and elastic
— keeping the vagina lubricated
— helping with concentration and reasoning
— enhancing magnesium uptake and improving insulin

Causes of Imbalance

Too much oestrogen can leave us oestrogen dominant. Oestrogen that is unobstructed by progesterone decreases libido, increases PMS and can increase the chances of fibrocystic breasts, fibroids in the uterus and oestrogen-driven cancers.

Progesterone decline is not the only reason for this. Elevated insulin increases the conversion of testosterone to oestrogen due to elevating aromatase activity, but SHBG also binds free oestrogen – elevated insulin and decreased SHBG mean more circulating free oestrogen.

Obesity and excess fat, especially around the middle, known as visceral adipose tissue (VAT), will produce its own oestrogen. (Just as with VAT in everyday life, the more we have the more we pay…) Obesity also increases inflammation in the body, leading to further conversion of oestrogen.

Constipation and impaired detoxification is another cause – our liver needs to package up the used oestrogen to get it ready to be removed via our stools. Increased stress, xeno-oestrogens, environmental toxins, as well as alcohol and caffeine consumption can also elevate oestrogen.

Causes of low oestrogen include:
— taking the Pill
— hysterectomy

Oestrogen and the Menopause

The main natural cause of low oestrogen is menopause, as the ovaries stop producing oestrogen but the adrenal glands continue producing it in peripheral tissue, such as brain, fat and skin. It is, however, becoming more prevalent in younger women, too. In premenopausal women, oestrogen production can become erratic, with surges of high levels alternating with periods of low levels.

— cancer treatment, such as chemotherapy and radiotherapy
— genetic diseases
— thyroid problems
— anorexia nervosa

Results of Imbalance

— mood swings
— memory loss
— problems focusing
— irregular/painful periods
— vaginal dryness
— irritability
— fatigue
— hot flushes
— night sweats
— stress
— anxiety
— loss of bone density
— depression
— breast tenderness
— PMS
— endometriosis
— weight gain
— infertility

Remedies

We need relatively small amounts of oestrogen to have an action in the body, which increases the need for tight control through lifestyle and dietary measures, and keeping an eye on the toxins we are exposed to. All Six Pillars are really important for oestrogen (*see* pages 60–81).

Cortisol
– the life saver

Cortisol, often known as the 'stress hormone', originates from the adrenal glands – small but mighty glands that sit above the kidneys. It's one of the hormones that we tend to produce more of as we age. It has a number of important functions, playing a role in:

— balancing blood sugar
— weight control
— the immune system
— stress reaction
— restful sleep
— mood

The adrenal glands respond to the signal from the hypothalamus and produce adrenaline, cortisol and dehydroepiandrosterone (DHEA). As with everything, the body keeps a tight control – this control is referred to as the hypothalamic-pituitary-adrenal axis (HPA), and is basically our built-in stress-busting pathway… if we don't abuse it.

Causes of Imbalance

A number of factors can dysregulate normal cortisol levels, including depression, a poor diet and modern-day stressful lifestyles.

In prehistoric times, stress came mostly in the form of threats to our survival. Our bodies evolved to cope via a 'fight-or-flight' response, preparing us for immediate activity. The body shuts down everything that is not important in that moment (like digestion and secretion of sex hormones). This energy burst is short-lived: we either run for our life, or fight for our life. Then, once the threat and stress is over our bodies should have a chance to rest and go back to normal.

Ideally, this stress response would be activated only when actually necessary – an acute fight-or-flight situation. But we are now living in a state of constant stress with no time to recover. Our bodies can't differentiate between a work anxiety and being chased by a lion. This means we're overusing and abusing cortisol, and this has overwhelming hormonal and health implications.

Results of Imbalance

— impaired immunity
— osteoporosis risk
— elevated blood pressure
— raised cholesterol levels
— visceral adipose tissue (belly fat)
— dysregulated blood-sugar levels
— insulin resistance
— irregular and painful periods
— PMS
— fatigue/insomnia
— irritability/anxiety

We are discussing an imbalance in cortisol output not Addisons or Cushings disease which are life-threatening medical conditions.

Remedies

Stress is a major trigger for people to eat poorly, quit healthy lifestyle programmes, and smoke and drink to excess or practise substance abuse. **If stress is a major player for you, look in detail at addressing Pillar Three: Nurture (*see* pages 68–71).**

Cortisol is necessary for life: it gets us up in the morning and gets us out of danger when necessary with the 'fight-or flight' response

Sleep Cycles

These days, our circadian rhythm – our natural body clock – is often out of kilter, and cortisol is very sensitive to this. Cortisol levels naturally rise in the mornings and drop in the evenings. As cortisol drops, melatonin, our sleep hormone, rises. So it follows that if our body clocks are in chaos, our cortisol levels will be, too.

How well do you sleep? Are you guilty of spending hours on your phone, iPad or watching TV till gone midnight? We know the blue light emitted by electronic devices can mess with our circadian rhythms and hormone levels.

In addition, we are not outside as much as we used to be, so we are not exposed to enough natural light and sunlight. Going outside during daylight hours is important, as there is a part of the brain that needs regular daylight stimulation to maintain circadian rhythms.

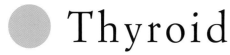 Thyroid

– the metabolism queen

The thyroid gland is a small butterfly-shaped gland located in the front of the neck just below the Adam's apple. It produces thyroid hormones called thyroxine (T4), and triiodothyronine (T3). T4 is considered to be a pro-hormone because it is relatively inactive and needs to be converted to T3, mainly in the liver. T3 (either derived from T4 or secreted as T3) is much more potent and is the biologically active hormone that performs a regulatory function in almost every cell in the body, including the brain. The thyroid gland also produces calcitonin, a hormone that plays a role in calcium balance.

In order to achieve these results there is a tight control in place called the hypothalamic-pituitary-thyroid axis, or HPT axis. The messages come from the hypothalamus, which secretes thyrotropin-releasing hormone (TRH); this stimulates the pituitary to release thyroid-stimulating hormone (TSH), which in turn stimulates the release of thyroid hormones from the thyroid gland.

Thyroid hormones:
— stimulate different metabolic functions in the cells
— help us grow thick hair on our head
— give us energy
— regulate temperature
— help with ideal weight maintenance

Thyroid hormones can affect:
— our menstrual cycle
— pregnancy
— skin hydration
— brain development
— cholesterol levels
— digestion
— memory
— concentration
— blood-sugar balance

Causes of Imbalance

Millions of people worldwide are affected by thyroid dysfunction, and women are more susceptible.

Our thyroid is affected by our environment, our lifestyle, our diet, inflammation, immune system dysregulation, toxins in the environment, digestive dysfunction and high stress levels. It's the perfect storm for a HPT dysfunction and its manifesting conditions, such as hypothyroidism (underactive thyroid), autoimmune conditions such as Hashimoto's, where your body's immune system cells attack your thyroid gland in error, and hyperthyroidism (overactive thyroid).

Results of Imbalance

— putting on weight or not
  being able to shift it
— feeling fatigued
— hair loss or thinning
— cold hands and feet
— feeling generally cold
— constipation
— elevated cholesterol
— irregular cycles
— miscarriage and other
  fertility issues
— brain fog that won't lift
— dysglycaemia/predisposition to
  insulin resistance

Note: hyperthyroidism can cause unexplained weight loss, shortness of breath without exertion, racing heart, muscle weakness, insomnia, loose stools, puffiness around the eyes and goitres (a swelling of the neck due to an enlarged thyroid gland). Always see your GP if you have any of these symptoms.

Remedies

If you're eating a nutrient-poor, low-fat diet, or one that lacks variety, and you are living a sedentary and stressful lifestyle, you're likely to be putting a strain on your thyroid. You can address these issues using the Six Pillars, especially Pillar One: Nourish, Pillar Two: Balance and Pillar Three: Nurture (*see* pages 60–71).

Proper Testing

If you ask your GP for a thyroid test, make sure you're getting a 'total thyroid screen' and not simply a TSH test. The latter doesn't give the whole picture, as it comes from the pituitary gland and not the thyroid.

An elevated TSH reading is an indication of thyroid hormone insufficiency and the pituitary's way of stepping up production. But just testing TSH is like looking at the tip of the iceberg.

Ideally, you need to test your free T4, free T3 and thyroid antibodies, including thyroid peroxidase (TPO) and anti-thyroglobulin antibodies. Adding a reverse T3 (rT3) test would be beneficial too – rT3 is like the brake that stops our thyroid hormone from working at the right time – it's a natural control measure. Unfortunately, toxins and inflammation can increase the levels of rT3, meaning that even if regular thyroid tests appear normal, high levels of rT3 could hinder our thyroid from working properly.

If your doctor can't do this level of testing, find a nutritional therapist or functional medical practioner who can.

Insulin

– the storage CEO

Insulin is created in the body to help regulate our blood-sugar levels. There always needs to be a certain level of sugar, otherwise known as glucose, circulating through our bloodstream at any given time for survival. Our body has very efficient self-regulating mechanisms, the main one being insulin, which is secreted by the pancreas in response to glucose in the bloodstream. Insulin is essential for regulating carbohydrate and fat metabolism; it takes the glucose from our blood and transports it into our cells so that it can be burned for energy, allowing blood sugar to return to its normal level. It prevents our blood sugar from getting too high, causing hyperglycaemia, which can prove fatal.

Causes of Imbalance

If we eat too many processed, sugary and refined carb foods our cells don't need all this glucose right away; insulin then carries the excess glucose to the liver (and muscles), where it is stored in a kind of 'reserve tank' in the form of glycogen. This can then be burned as fuel when we need it, between meals and during exercise, for example. If you regularly eat too much sugar, the tank fills up and the excess glucose is converted to fatty acids (triglycerides/fat). This fat is stored in your adipose tissue (fat cells) and you will mainly see it deposited around the waist – enter VAT, the dreaded muffin top.

What else causes this insulin reaction?
— eating foods high in refined carbohydrates and sugar
— eating or drinking stimulants like caffeine or fizzy drinks
— stress
— skipping meals
— excessive weight
— hormonal conditions
— sedentary lifestyle or inactivity
— toxins in the environment
— insomnia
— smoking
— endocrine-disrupting chemicals
— inflammation

Results of Imbalance

Regular peaks and troughs in blood sugar (dysglycaemia) eventually take their toll. Your body may become so sensitive to changes in blood sugar that excess insulin is released, making blood-sugar levels crash below normal and causing hypoglycaemia. So instead of feeling energized, with noticeable improvements in mental capacity and emotional wellbeing, and feeling satisfied for hours after eating, you are left feeling hyper, agitated, angry or irritable, low or depressed and tired. Thyroid disorders can further add to dysglycaemia by slowing glucose uptake as well as the response of insulin.

Dysglycaemia in turn stimulates the release of cortisol from the adrenal glands in order to break down blood-sugar stores in a bid to raise your blood levels again. Our pancreas responds by pumping out even more insulin in its bid to keep us alive; these high insulin levels are referred to as hyperinsulinemia.

Over time, the insulin receptors have an impaired sensitivity to the hormone insulin – leading to what's called insulin resistance – leaving you with both elevated blood sugar and insulin in the bloodstream, which is dangerous for your health. Insulin resistance is a precursor for Type 2 diabetes and exacerbates hormonal conditions such as PCOS.

Remedies

Each of the other five of our Sassy Six are intrinsically linked with insulin. We have seen how the thyroid can affect insulin and how insulin can increase aromatase and decrease SHBG, which in turn affects both oestrogen and testosterone. It has a very close relationship with cortisol and therefore can affect all of the Sassy Six hormones, including progesterone and thyroid. So Pillar Two: Balance is key, but all Six Pillars (see pages 60–81) have a part to play in keeping insulin regulated.

Sugar is the wrinkle monster!

The Sweet Stuff

Sugar is well and truly in the media spotlight and has opened many great conversations in recent years. It's the ingredient I'm asked most about in my clinic, and the one most people fear parting with. The world over, we're succumbing to so many of its effects. The rate of Type 2 diabetes in the UK, for example, has increased by 60 per cent over the past decade, and we are starting to see it more in young children because of poor diet and a sedentary lifestyle. This is one habit you're going to have to break.

Still not convinced? Sugar is the wrinkle monster! It binds to the skin's collagen causing its fibres to stick together and become rigid; creating wrinkles, sags and bags. This elevated inflammation also stimulates the breakdown of collagen and elastin (the support structures that keep our skin plump and juicy) resulting in sagging skin and further wrinkles.

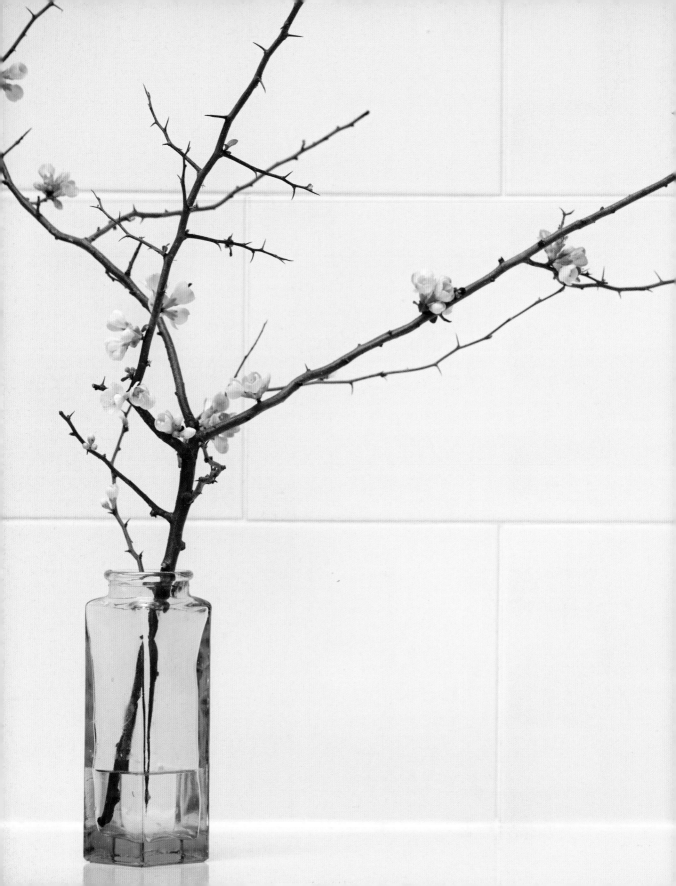

PART 2

showstoppers

What's Your Dis-ease?

We are experiencing high levels of menstrual and reproductive 'dis-ease'. There's a worrying incidence of everything from endometriosis, polycystic ovary syndrome (PCOS) and fibroids to cysts, PMS, cramps, heavy bleeding, subfertility, miscarriage and pelvic pain.
If conversations in clinic and among friends are anything to go by, all these conditions seem to be on the rise. We need to get back in balance.

The 'Average' Cycle

Although 28 days is referred to as an 'average cycle', not all cycles are the same. So try not to stress if yours is 25 days or 35 days or it changes from month to month. We are so biochemically individual that our cycle can vary from one woman to another, and from one cycle to the next. Only approximately 40 per cent of the menstruating women I see in my clinic have a 28-day cycle.

I recommend downloading a period tracker app. It's a really easy way to log your cycles, symptoms and spot patterns. It will help you track the date of your next period, your likely fertile dates and ovulation and, most importantly, to know what's normal for you.

Tune in to Your Hormones

The male and female bodies may both be ruled by hormones, but it's only us women who have to cope with radical hormonal changes throughout our lives: puberty and starting our periods, pregnancy, postpartum, breastfeeding, perimenopause, and the grand finale, menopause. A lot of the time these changes go hand in hand with uncomfortable issues – persistent symptoms that need to be addressed, ideally understanding and rectifying the underlying cause.

Empowerment starts with understanding. I encourage you to take the first steps by tuning in. Our bodies give us clues, often in the form of little niggles – a change in a cycle, pain, mood swings, cravings – that suggest something is going on. How would you feel if these symptoms only happened every now and again instead of being the norm? This book is an invitation to notice how your body talks to you, and to pay attention before the niggles become symptoms you can't ignore.

What's Stopping the Show?

In Part 1 (see pages 14–31), we looked at our endocrine system's harmonic symphony and our monthly cycle's Viennese waltz. We learned about our Sassy Six and how, when they're all working in harmony, we should be

It's OK, I'm on the Pill

When it's used correctly and for what it was designed to do (to prevent a pregnancy) the contraceptive pill can have its advantages, not least liberation. In many cases, however, it is prescribed to reduce period pain or PMS, 'fix' an irregular cycle, deal with acne or symptoms of PCOS and endometriosis. It can work, but it's important to realize it's just a sticking plaster. Taking the Pill masks symptoms and gives you a false 'period' (or no period at all if you take packets back to back as many women do). Unfortunately, if you have not dealt with the underlying causes of your hormonal imbalances, when you come off the Pill the symptoms will come back and with a vengeance.

Side Effects to be Aware of:

— **Nutrient deficiencies.** Taking the Pill for many years can leave us with deficiencies including B vitamins, vitamin C, selenium, magnesium and zinc. All are needed for healthy functioning of the thyroid, immune system, adrenal glands and liver.

— **Disruption of the microbiome.** The Pill can disrupt our gut microbes, which can lead to the overgrowth of harmful bacteria and yeast. This can leave us constipated as well as plagued by chronic yeast infections like candida, while further reducing nutrient absorption.

— **Mood changes and mood swings.** The Pill is associated with depression. All too often doctors overlook this, instead writing a prescription for antidepressant drugs – another sticking plaster.

— **Reduced sex drive.** The Pill increases sex hormone binding globulin (SHBG), which in turn can lower testosterone, leading to a lower libido. It can also affect thyroid hormones, potentially leading to weight gain, insomnia and further constipation.

— **Inflammation.** Studies have linked the Pill to chronic inflammation and increased insulin sensitivity.

able to sit back and enjoy the show. All too often, however, the show gets interrupted. Our hormones aren't in balance, the dance isn't happening and the symphony is off key. There are lots of potential 'showstoppers',

from the conditions and symptoms listed opposite and above to environmental or dietary factors. We take a closer look at them – and what we can do about them – in this section. The show must go on!

Premenstrual Syndrome (PMS)

When Bad Moods Happen to Good Women

Although PMS doesn't cause a hormonal imbalance, it can feel like it's stopping the show. You will notice that many hormonal imbalances come with mood swings, irritability and anger. I'm sure we've all been there – one minute we're all sweetness and light, the next we're like fire-breathing dragons.

PMS is a complex syndrome of physical and psychological symptoms. They can occur anything from a few days to two weeks before your period, so that can be as much as half the month feeling less than your best. Symptoms can vary from month to month in intensity and will improve once menstruation starts, so you can find yourself wishing for your period.

Many jokes are made about women and PMS, but it can be a hugely debilitating time. There are over 150 symptoms associated with PMS, including emotional, physical, cognitive and behavioural complaints. The intensity of the symptoms can be so severe that they cause social dysfunction and/or affect work performance – some women experience such significant and extreme symptoms that they are diagnosed with a condition called premenstrual dysphoric disorder (PMDD).

How Complicated is it?

In the 1980s, researcher Guy Abraham tried to create a classification of subgroups of PMS according to symptoms. He proposed four distinct groups:

PMS A	Anxiety, tension, irritability, anger, mood swings
PMS C	Food cravings, increased appetite, hypoglycaemia, fatigue, dizziness, headaches
PMS D	Decreased energy, depression, forgetfulness, emotionality, insomnia
PMS H	Abdominal bloating, oedema (swelling) of fingers/ankles, breast pain

While this classification highlights the many and varied symptoms involved in PMS, I'm not sure how helpful it is. If you regularly experience PMS, you're probably looking at it and thinking 'I have symptoms in more than one box'. And, in my experience, it's true that women rarely experience a symptom from only one subgroup. Although there is a wide spectrum of symptoms that are common hormonal patterns in women that have PMS, the complex interrelationships between our Sassy Six (*see* pages 20–31) mean our symptoms can be ever changing.

There are some truths, for example, low thyroid and elevated cortisol are common in PMS, as is elevated insulin from a high-sugar diet. But the takeaway message here is it's complicated – we're complicated – and the solution to PMS is not looking at individual symptoms but overall balance. Rest assured diet and lifestyle changes can have a huge, positive impact on your symptoms. Follow the Six Pillars on pages 60–81 and my four-week plan, and kiss goodbye to moods, bloating, cravings and more – hopefully for good.

Many jokes are made about women and PMS but it can be a hugely debilitating time. There are over 150 symptoms associated with PMS

What Else Might be Causing Your PMS?

— low thyroid
— high cortisol levels
— excess oestrogen
— low progesterone
— impaired liver function
— reduced serotonin (a result of gut dysbiosis)
— increased testosterone
— increased prolactin
— low vitamin B6 levels
— low magnesium levels
— a low-fat, high-sugar diet
— stress
— smoking and alcohol
— VAT

Toxins

Chemical Sisters

Never before have we been so bombarded by harmful chemicals on a daily basis. We're exposed to over 80,000 toxins circulating in our environment. Short of living in a glass bubble, we can't avoid them. And these substances, which may cause distress or disease to our bodies, can be found in everything from our food, water and soil to the air we breathe.

Our modern diet of fast foods full of refined carbohydrates, sugar, artificial sweeteners, high-fructose syrups, caffeine and trans fats places an extra burden on our detoxification pathways, even more so if food has been smothered with pesticides and insecticides. The non-organic meat products we eat come with a host of added extras, such as synthetic hormones and antibiotics.

The environment is full of toxins in the form of cleaning materials, pharmaceutical drugs, car fumes, factory by-products, non-stick cookware, plastic food containers, candles, air fresheners and more. We're surrounded by chemical toxins and heavy metals such as lead, mercury, cadmium, arsenic, nickel and aluminium, which can have serious health implications if they start to build up in our bodies.

Make-up and other cosmetic beauty products can contain hormone-altering chemicals, including parabens and phthalates. Think of all the products you apply to your face daily.

Love Your Liver

The liver is one of the major organs responsible for removing harmful substances from the body, so that they cannot damage our DNA, hormones and nerve-signalling processes and cell structure. These can be internal by-products of metabolism (carbon dioxide, spent hormones, ammonia, urea, lactic acid, rancid

How Do Chemicals Affect Our Hormones?

Pesticides, bisphenol A (BPA), phthalates and other chemicals very often have endocrine-disrupting properties. They artificially increase levels of hormones in the body, or impede their proper and essential breakdown. This also puts a lot of stress on our liver. These synthetic chemicals may be carcinogens (cancer causing) or even obesogens, which disrupt normal fat metabolism and can lead to obesity (*see* my Top Four Foes on page 40).

Your skin is your largest organ, so treat it with love and care, and eliminate toxins. Also see page 75 for more tips on being a smart label reader.

fats, by-products of microbial imbalance in the gut), or any of the external substances already listed.

Liver Health is Crucial for:
— a strong immune system
— a balanced inflammatory function
— a well-regulated endocrine function
— a healthy neurological system
— a strong musculoskeletal system
— abundant cellular energy production
— an overall sense of wellbeing

Although the liver is a very adaptive organ and can handle a lot of damage before showing signs of disease, a poorly functioning or overburdened liver can have knock-on effects on the rest of the body. How the liver works (in very simple terms) is by filtering the blood so that any harmful toxins are recognized and are then sent through a series of pathways to make them either harmless or more toxic, to prepare them for excretion out of the body. Unfortunately, we can load toxins in faster than our liver can eliminate them. So our liver is busy dealing with everything we keep throwing at it instead of with jobs like the proper metabolism and elimination of oestrogen, for example. Caffeine, alcohol, xeno-oestrogens, high sugar, low fibre and low nutrients all put a strain on this organ.

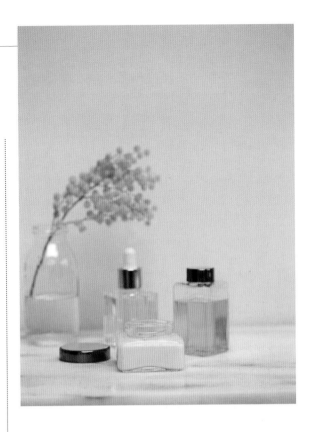

The good news is you don't need to follow a restrictive 'detox' regime to love your liver and balance your hormones. My four-week plan and Pillar Four: Cleanse (see pages 72–75) are designed to support your liver on a daily basis

Toxin Watch – My Top Four Foes

Xeno-oestrogens are oestrogen-mimicking chemicals. They are man-made environmental compounds that have a strong oestrogenic effect in the body, so their presence in the body may lead to negative effects on the reproductive system, through disruption of the hormonal balance necessary for proper functioning. Xeno-oestrogens can dock onto our oestrogen receptors, affect thyroid function and even our central nervous system. Our body thinks, 'Great, there is a hormone here.' But they are impostors.

The really scary thing is that they are found in thousands of everyday products, from plastic and metal food containers to detergents, flame retardants, toys, cosmetics and paint. They've even been found in drinking water, probably from the synthetic oestrogen consumed by women taking the contraceptive pill (not filtered out by the water recycling process). And once inside us, they can build up in the body. Xeno-oestrogens are lipophilic, meaning they are stored in fat tissue and have carcinogenic potential, increasing our risk of some cancers such as breast cancer. It's even thought that these oestrogen imposters are potentially contributing to the early onset of puberty, sometimes in girls as young as eight.

1. **Parabens**, which are found in lotions, sun creams and moisturisers, are used to preserve the lotions and help them penetrate the skin. Unfortunately, they are a xeno-oestrogen and they have been linked to infertility and breast cancer.

2. **Phthalates** are used in soft, flexible plastics and in polyvinyl chloride (PVC) products. They are found in perfumes, nail polish, shampoos, soap, hairspray, shower curtains, baby toys, vinyl flooring and car interiors. They have been shown to bind chemicals together and impact on the hormonal system by affecting testosterone and SHBG, and blocking oestrogen production, leading to ovulation and fertility issues. In addition, they have been linked to cancer, obesity, Type 2 diabetes, allergies/asthma and ADHD.

3. **Bisphenol-A (BPA)** is a polycarbonate plastic widely used in reusable water bottles, baby bottles, dummies, plastic utensils, children's toys, the lining of many cans of food, certain microwaveable and reusable plastic containers, even thermal paper receipts. We are surrounded by the stuff! BPA has a 'leaky' nature and, over time, can leach from plastic bottles, cans and plastic vacuum packs into our food, especially when the plastic is heated or as it ages. It's thought to be more easily absorbed by fatty foods. BPA is a known endocrine-disrupting hormone and it slows down our thyroid function by blocking thyroid receptors. It is also linked to cancer, obesity and infertility. Luckily, it is now possible to source BPA-free bottles and canned products.

4. **Dioxins** are compounds known as persistent environmental pollutants (POPs). They are released into the atmosphere when materials like PVC are burned, and from other waste materials and industrial processes. They're produced during the manufacture of pesticides and herbicides, the bleaching of pulp and paper, and are found in some tampons and sanitary towels. Dioxins can also be a result of natural processes, and volcanoes and forest fires release them into the air. They can accumulate in the food chain, mainly in the fatty tissue of animals, and we eat them in meat and dairy products, fish and shellfish. Dioxins are endocrine disruptors and can cause reproductive and developmental problems, as well as damage the immune system.

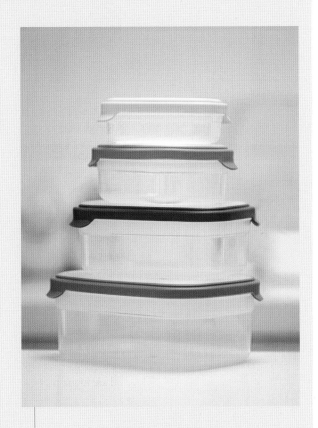

Let's face it, it's not always possible to avoid plastic. However, you can still love your hormones by choosing BPA-free products, such as these storage boxes, and avoiding foods wrapped in plastic.

So What's the Solution?

Yes, it's a chemical world – but it's not all doom and gloom. As we become more aware of the health implications, many companies have moved away from using these chemicals in response to consumer demand.

You can buy organic beauty products, personal-care items and environmentally friendly household cleaners. And it's fairly easy to buy less packaged food and choose glass, metal and wooden kitchen implements and storage.

There are fantastic resources out there to check what chemicals a product might contain – look up the Environmental Working Group, the Soil Association database and Turning Green, for starters.

Don't be taken in by buzz words like 'all natural' and 'pure' – these aren't regulated terms (unlike organic) and are no substitute for careful checking of the label.

Don't be taken in by buzz words like 'all natural' and 'pure' – these aren't regulated terms

The Modern Diet

Our Complex Relationship with Food

Eating has become a gratifying pursuit, and cooking merely a hobby. So often, we don't have time – or rather don't make the time – to cook real food. We grab something to microwave (in plastic), a processed, convenience food. But our bodies don't care how busy we are, they're still hard-wired for food as nature intended it: clean, unprocessed and whole.

Optimum nutrition is an important first step in any hormone-rebalancing programme. The body needs specific vitamins, minerals and fatty acids to produce sex hormones as well as stress hormones. Our hormones also need to be nourished to keep us slim, energized, balanced and mentally sharp. What you put on the end of your fork matters.

When Good Food Goes Bad

Dietary stresses are a major contributor to female hormonal imbalance. This can be consuming the wrong foods, over-eating or skipping meals – things we all do occasionally without realizing the adverse effect on our hormones. Obesity also has a negative effect on hormonal balance.

And it's a confusing business. For example, you might think favouring a low-fat diet is the key to losing weight and staying healthy. But I believe this dietary trend has been one of the biggest causes of health issues today. Fat and cholesterol are important building blocks needed for the production of sex hormones. Eating low-fat reduces your ability to make sex hormones and it also strips you of essential, fat-soluble nutrients like vitamins A, D, E and K. And let's be honest, if 'fat-free' worked we would all be super-healthy and within our ideal body-weight range.

Waist Away

Struggling to lose that belly fat? I hear you. I've been there, done that and couldn't fit into the T-shirt. The solution? Stop looking at the scales. We are no longer interested in weight. I want you to think of 'waist loss' not weight loss. Our weight naturally fluctuates throughout the month. Inches lost, especially around the middle, are a more accurate indicator that fat is coming off and staying off.

What's Making us Weight-loss Resistant?

Have you looked in the mirror lately and noticed an extra band around your middle, the dreaded bulge that won't shift? The tummy you have to tuck into your trousers? Many women say they've tried everything and just can't seem to slim down. They may think they're making all the right changes, but they're resistant to weight loss. Yes, excessive eating, inappropriate portion sizes and inactivity definitely play a part. But there is so much more to it than that. We have already seen that an imbalance in the Sassy Six can lead to weight gain. Excess oestrogen, insulin, cortisol and impaired thyroid function all have a major impact on the storage and increase of fat around the middle.

Nutrition is the foundation of good health and balanced hormones. Weight loss, if you need it, will be the result

Sleep Less, Weigh More?

It's true, poor sleep patterns can lead to weight gain. How? Because sleep is important for the control of insulin, leptin and ghrelin – hormones that work together to control feelings of hunger, cravings and satiety (fullness). Leptin is produced in adipose (fat) cells – it signals to the hypothalamus when we have enough energy/are full and increases metabolism. It's at its highest after a meal, when it tells the hypothalamus we have had enough and should reduce food intake. Ghrelin is produced in the gastrointestinal tract and stimulates appetite – I like to think of ghrelin as a gremlin, because poor sleep reduces levels of leptin and increases ghrelin levels, meaning you don't feel satisfied after you eat and your appetite is stimulated. Gremlins always want more!

Chronic Stress

Are Modern Lifestyles to Blame?

We've talked about cortisol, our stress hormone, and how stress continues to be the biggest crisis facing women's health in the 21st century. Our bodies were designed to buffer small bursts of acute stress very intermittently. They were not built to deal with the chronic daily stress that the majority of us now seem to be under.

Today, despite not being faced with the same dangers as our ancestors, our bodies go through the same physiological changes when we are stressed. When our adrenal glands send out adrenaline and cortisol these messengers override any other function in the body. Plus, these stress hormones change the way our bodies work. You see, when we enter this fight-or-flight response, we activate the autonomic nervous system (ANS). The ANS is responsible for the regulation of certain body processes, such as blood pressure, heart rate and rate of breathing. The ANS has two main divisions: sympathetic and parasympathetic.

The sympathetic division is activated in emergencies that cause us stress and require us to 'fight' or take 'flight'; it uses a lot of energy, our blood pressure increases, our heart beats faster, lungs breathe deeper to allow more oxygen to spread through the body, more nutrition for brain and muscles is utilized, blood-sugar stores are broken down to free up more energy, our arteries widen to allow more blood to pump through. We are on alert, focused, ready to go. The sympathetic ANS will also shut down systems that we don't need – like reproduction, hunger, growth, digestion.

The parasympathetic ANS, activated in non-emergencies, allows us to 'rest' and 'digest'. It conserves and restores, promotes growth, repair and sleep, builds tissues and ensures proper functioning of hormones while it stimulates the digestive tract to process food and eliminate waste efficiently.

Stress on the Brain?

Have you noticed that your memory is not what it used to be? One of the effects of chronic over-exposure to cortisol is that it can affect the frontal cortex in your brain. The stress response, designed to help us survive at all costs, starts in our brain. When it's activated, it can affect your memory and your ability to learn. So, if you're having brain fog or feeling forgetful, you could be succumbing to stress.

In prehistoric times stress never lasted long, and because it invariably resulted in physical activity (think of outrunning that lion), glucose was quickly metabolized, bringing blood-sugar levels back to normal. This meant that stress hormones were quickly rebalanced. Not so with the chronic stress we're under today. No wonder our hormones aren't happy. But Pillar Three: Nurture (*see* pages 68–71) and Pillar Six: Restore (*see* pages 78–81) are designed to address stress once and for all.

Inflammation – the Internal Fire

Inflammation is an important part of our immune system response. When we have a sore throat or an insect bite, our immune system jumps into action – the area is swollen, red and hot from an increase of blood flow as white blood cells rush to the area. Our adrenal hormones interact with the immune system and trigger an inflammatory release. This would make evolutionary sense; you need inflammation in case you get hurt by that lion chasing you. But chronic stress means your immune system is constantly, unnecessarily active. This has a knock-on effect on hormonal health, and low-level chronic inflammation is at the root of countless illnesses, from allergies, autoimmune diseases and heart disease to obesity, diabetes, dementia, depression, asthma, psoriasis and even cancer.

Your Adrenal Bank Account

We might not be able to eliminate stress from our lives, but we can make sure we've got enough reserves in our wellbeing fund to protect us when stress comes along. Just remember, this adrenal bank account has no overdraft or credit card facility – if you go overdrawn you'll feel terrible, so try to keep everything in balance.

Withdrawals:
— poor diet
— not enough sleep
— not enough or too much physical activity
— chronic, unrelenting stress

Deposits:
— rest
— meditation
— moderate exercise
— yoga
— nourishing food
— me time
— sleep
— laughter
— love

Poor Elimination

Optimize Your Gut Function

How is your digestion? We don't always like to talk about our tummies or, worse still, our toilet habits. But it really matters. Having terrible digestive complaints, not pooing for days or passing stools that aren't formed are all signs that something isn't right with your digestion. This can have a spill-over effect on hormonal balance. Gut irritability, if left unchecked, can lead to the development of a whole host of health conditions and create additional stress, inflammation and hormonal imbalance in the body. Many of the hormonal conditions that I treat in my clinic are connected to a problem with the digestive system. Often, people don't understand the crucial link between a healthy digestive system, brain and optimally functioning hormones. Getting your digestion in good working order needs to become a priority.

Gut-brain?

We all know that feeling of butterflies in the stomach, or suddenly having cramps and rushing to the loo before a big event. There's a definite connection between your digestive system and your emotions. It's called the gut-brain axis, and it explains terms like 'gut feeling' and 'gut instinct'.

Your digestive system has its own independent nervous system, called the enteric nervous system (ENS), which communicates with our brain and is connected via the autonomic nervous system (ANS) – the sympathetic and parasympathetic nerves. That means that stress has an effect on this system too.

A very important task of the ENS is to keep everything moving from the top down, which is done through the contraction of muscle cells (peristalsis). As the microbiome (gut flora) makes certain vitamins and absorbs our nutrients, the ENS aids digestion by triggering gut hormones and enzymes, while keeping the blood flowing to move the absorbed food and nutrients to where they need to go. It also plays a role in immune and inflammatory processes in the body by communicating with these cells in the gut.

The digestive system forms the basis of our immune system, as around 60 per cent of our immune system lies right under the one-cell-layer-thick lining of our gut. It's also where the majority of our neurotransmitters (brain chemicals) like serotonin (aka the happy hormone) originate. It's important that we keep this system happy so that we can feel happy – a happy gut is a happy brain.

Meet Your Microbiome

The microbiome is the collective name for our internal ecosystem of gut microbes. These trillions of microbes live in our intestine (gut) where they help us digest food, absorb nutrients, produce vitamins, regulate hormones, fluff out our stools and excrete toxins. We need to nourish them so they can keep on doing these vital jobs.

Everyone's microbiome is unique and there are hundreds of different strains of bacteria that can inhabit it. We know that a healthy microbiome is diverse and abundant, and we can keep it that way with a diverse diet rich in whole foods, prebiotics and probiotics (my 'eco warriors'). An unbalanced or limited microbiome can allow 'bad' microbes like parasites, unfavourable bacteria and yeasts such as candida to proliferate. Too many of the wrong bacteria can cause an imbalance called gut or bacterial 'dysbiosis' and lead to serious damage to your health. This bacterial dybiosis can increase an enzyme called beta-glucuronidase, which can actually break the bond between the packaged ready-to-be-excreted oestrogen that the liver worked so hard on, causing it to recirculate.

We can implement simple and achievable strategies for good gut health in Pillar Two: Balance (*see* pages 64–67).

What Are You Popping?

Do you poo every day? And if so, is it hard, like little pellets? Or is it runny, like water, or soft, like cow dung? Does it hurt to pass, causing you to bleed on the way out? Have a look at the poo chart on the following page and see where you fit in.

WARNING: it gets a bit graphic on the next page

Healthy Pooing

The gut has a very important gatekeeper role – let only the good stuff in (nutrients, vitamins and minerals, good bacteria) and keep the bad stuff out (undigested food, toxins, bad bacteria). If this important role is compromised in any way, we start to feel the effects of absorbing toxins, reacting to foods. It can trigger an autoimmune reaction, cause bloating, excessive gas and cramps, fatigue, and all sorts of pooing problems, which hinder proper elimination of all the packaged-up hormones that need to find the exit. What can cause this? You guessed it: a diet high in sugar and processed junk foods, low in vegetables and fibre. The overuse of antibiotics, anti-inflammatories such as painkillers and, of course, our chronic stress won't help either.

Poo Chart (we've kept it as clean as we can!)

TYPE 1		**Small, separate, solid pieces (almost like droppings), which are hard to pass**
		A clear indication that you are constipated. Are you eating enough vegetables and drinking enough water?
TYPE 2		**Lumpy sausage, which is hard to pass**
		An indication that you are slightly constipated or heading that way.
TYPE 3		**Sausage with cracked surface**
		A near-perfect poo, but the cracked surface could indicate that you are dehydrated.
TYPE 4		**Silky-smooth soft sausage, easy to pass**
		Ta-da! The perfect poo.
TYPE 5		**Small, separate, soft pieces**
		A loose, soft stool can indicate a lack of fibre in the diet.
TYPE 6		**Mushy with little or no form**
		Could be an indication of inflammation of the bowel, low eco-warriors, that you are eating something that doesn't agree with you or that you are heading for diarrhoea.
TYPE 7		**Completely watery**
		A clear indication that you have diarrhoea, not something you should have every day.

Chart adapted from the Bristol Stool Scale (Heaton et al, 1992)

Don't Hold it In!

Everyone's digestion differs according to what we've eaten or what's going on in our lives. But, on balance, most of your stools should be Type 4s. Type 1 is constipation and Type 7 is diarrhoea – problems we all experience from time to time, but which shouldn't be a daily occurrence.

Having days between bowel movements is bad news for hormones, and is possibly caused by a hormonal imbalance. Constipation is not normal, no matter what your age. In fact, it worsens existing hormonal imbalances because your body cannot excrete excess oestrogen. When this happens, oestrogen is reabsorbed, recirculated and dumped back into our bloodstream through the gut. This is after our superhero liver has done the work to get rid of it in the first place.

I'm confident that my Balance Plan will help sort your elimination issues and help you alleviate that digestive discomfort. But if you still feel you're not going to the loo enough, or too much, or what's coming out isn't right, ask your GP to investigate issues such as irritable bowel syndrome (IBS). Any persistent change in bowel habits that's not normal for you should always be reported to your doctor.

Eat your way to Better Gut Health

Constipation is not 'normal' – but neither is pooing five times a day. If you are having tummy troubles, we need to sort them out. Reassessing your diet is the perfect place to start.

The following recipes are all included in my four-week meal plan and are particularly good for digestion:
— the green smoothies (*see* pages 109 and 110)
— Tropical Turmeric Smoothie (*see* page 108)
— Spiced Matcha Latte (*see* page 112)
— Raw Oat, Fruit & Nut Porridge (*see* page 114)
— Quinoa & Berry Porridge (*see* page 116)
— Chicken Stock (*see* page 166)
— Steamed Spring Greens (*see* page 196)
— Steamed Greens (*see* page 198)
— Mixed Herb Salad (*see* page 191)
— Simple Sauerkraut (*see* page 200)

PCOS & Endometriosis

As we've seen, there are lots of Showstoppers that can prevent our hormones from functioning optimally. But if you have a gynaecological condition it can feel like there's nothing you can do to regain control and bring some balance to your hormonal life.

First of all, let me say that any unusual pain, bleeding, discomfort, lumps or anything that isn't normal for you should always be reported to your GP. And if any of the symptoms described on these pages sound familiar, ask your doctor to investigate. This book isn't designed to be a medical guide and there are many more gynaecological issues you may face. Here I'm going to look at just two of the most common: polycystic ovarian syndrome, or PCOS, and endometriosis. While there's no quick fix for these conditions and you may need medication, you can make a big difference through diet and lifestyle changes. Work with a qualified nutritionist on a personal plan tailored to you.

Polycystic Ovary Syndrome (PCOS)

This hormonal disorder causes a collection of cysts to form around the outer edge of the ovaries. It's not just the ovaries that are affected; PCOS causes hormonal imbalance in all your body's glands, including the pituitary, pineal, thyroid, parathyroid, thymus, adrenal and pancreas. Researchers are not sure of the precise cause, but we know this condition causes the ovaries to produce higher than normal amounts of testosterone, which can interfere with egg production and increase the risk of miscarriage. Many researchers believe PCOS is caused by excessive amounts of insulin being produced in the body. Excess insulin leads to insulin resistance, which then prompts the ovaries to produce extra testosterone, resulting in many of the symptoms associated with PCOS.

Five to ten per cent of women may have PCOS – I am one of them and know the heartache it can cause

What are Some of the Symptoms?

— oily skin
— recurring acne
— infrequent, irregular periods or amenorrhea (no periods)
— painful periods
— difficulty or inability to get pregnant due to irregular or lack of ovulation
— hirsutism – excess hair growth on the face and body
— weight gain, especially around the middle
— hair loss from the head, or thinning hair
— skin tags, typically in the armpit or neck area
— low levels of sex hormone binding globulin (SHBG)
— recurrent miscarriage
— high prolactin and high levels of oestrogen
— heavy periods, with a lot of clotting

Conventional Treatment for PCOS

— medication to help regulate your periods, such as a low-dose birth control pill
— metformin is commonly prescribed to regulate insulin for women with insulin resistance and Type 2 diabetes
— for those wanting to become pregnant, a medication such as Clomid (Clomifene citrate) will help induce ovulation
— medication to reduce excess hair growth

So What Can we Do?

PCOS may be a lifetime condition, but I can't stress enough what a massive help improving your diet and lifestyle can be – I am living proof of that. We need to be looking at correcting the underlying causes of PCOS, which means correcting insulin resistance and eating to nourish the body (*see* the recipe section on pages 106–213) and balance the Sassy Six hormones (explored in detail on pages 20–31). Even if you need to take the conventional route, please work on the underlying causes by taking this holistic approach and following the Balance Plan (especially Pillar Two: Balance, *see* pages 64–67) at the same time.

You Are Not Alone

It's thought five to ten per cent of women may have PCOS – I am one of them and know the heartache it can cause – but many may remain undiagnosed. Symptoms vary between women and it can be hard to pinpoint, but if you recognize several of the signs or symptoms listed, do see your GP for further investigation.

Endometriosis

Endometriosis is a common condition in which endometrial tissue (often referred to as endometrial implants) is found outside the womb. Endometriosis affects two million women in the UK and is said to be an autoimmune condition. It commonly occurs between the ages of 25 and 40 in menstruating women, but can also occur at a younger age. It's rare post menopause.

Endometrial growths most commonly develop around the ovaries, fallopian tubes, the lining of the abdomen, and on the bowel or bladder. What happens is the endometrium still responds to the hormonal fluctuations associated with the menstrual cycle, so it thickens, breaks down and bleeds, just as your womb lining does each month if you don't fall pregnant. But whereas your womb lining has somewhere to go and you lose it as menstrual blood, the blood in endometriosis becomes trapped, irritating local tissue, causing pain and inflammation.

What are Some of the Symptoms?

The key symptoms include painful menstruation (dysmenorrhea), heavy periods, pain in the lower abdomen, pelvis or lower back, painful intercourse (dyspareunia), bleeding between periods and infertility or difficulty conceiving. Other symptoms may include discomfort with urination and/or bowel movements, bleeding from the nose, bladder or bowels, coughing blood, nausea, fainting, and lethargy.

Some women don't have any symptoms from endometriosis and may not find out they have the condition until they have trouble getting pregnant and some investigation is done.

Conventional Treatment for Endometriosis

Your GP may refer you to a gynaecologist who may do an internal examination and ultrasound scan. For a definitive diagnosis to be made, a laparoscopy (a fibre-optic viewing tube) in the abdominal area and a biopsy need to be carried out under general anaesthetic.

There is no absolute cure for endometriosis, so treatment is based around easing the symptoms, shrinking or slowing down the endometrial tissue growth and, where possible, preserving or restoring fertility. This is achieved through a combination of anti-inflammatory pain relief, hormone treatment, the Pill or surgery.

So What Can we Do?

High levels of inflammation and oestrogen activity are associated with endometriosis. So there's much we can do to address these, namely balancing blood sugar, maintaining a healthy body weight, reducing inflammation and exposure to environmental toxins, supporting elimination and keeping active. The Balance Plan can help you with them all.

High levels of inflammation and oestrogen are associated with endometriosis. Changing your diet and lifestyle can work wonders at alleviating symptoms, allowing you to flourish.

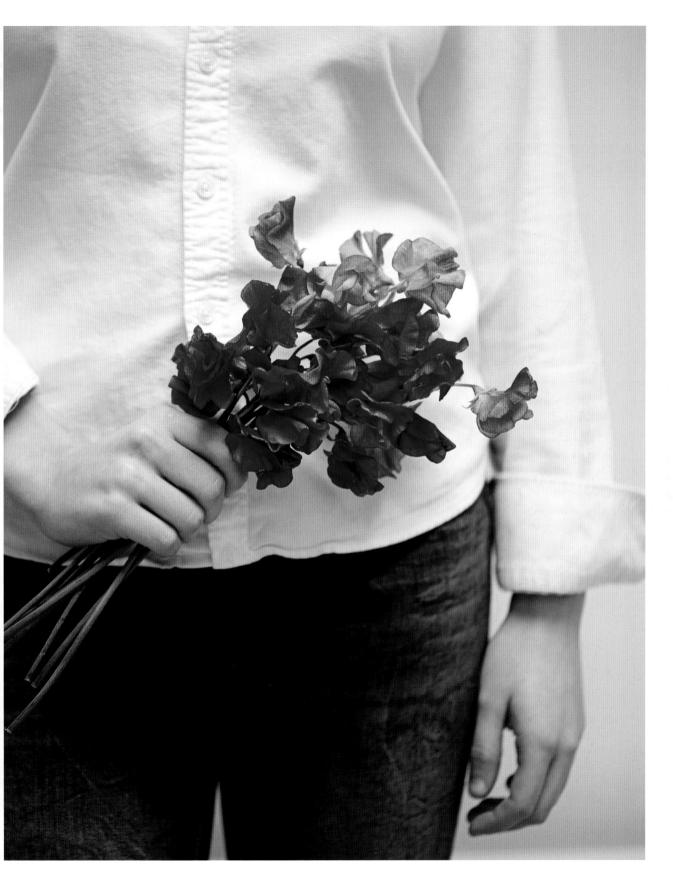

Perimenopause

Changing Times

The word 'menopause' conjures up different feelings. Some of us are filled with dread, viewing it as an illness or a sign of old age; some can't wait to finally stop menstruating. Menopause itself refers to your final period, and the average age for that in the UK is 51. The years leading up to it, a time of hormonal flux, are referred to as the perimenopause. But why do some women sail through this life stage and others feel like they have been hit by a ten-tonne truck?

So What's Going on, Exactly?

Let's get one thing straight. The menopause is not a disease or a medical condition. Menopause signifies a major transition in a woman's life: it's the end of the menstrual cycle as you reach the end of your natural reproductive life. Simply put, you've run out of eggs. How do you know when it's happened to you? If you've not had your period for a year, your doctor will say you've been through the menopause.

Perimenopause describes the years leading up to that. And for some women symptoms can start to show themselves as many as 10 to 15 – yes 15 – years before it's all over (others are symptom free or only notice a couple of symptoms in their late 40s, so don't panic and assume it's going to be awful). Over the years, the number of eggs in our ovaries becomes depleted and the functionality of our ovaries decreases. With these changes come reduced oestrogen, progesterone and testosterone. The adrenal glands and fat cells take over the production of sex hormones, so we are not totally losing our Sassy Six. As these hormone levels start to drop, the normal menstrual cycle becomes distorted, eventually stopping completely.

Possible Symptoms of Perimenopause
— hot flushes
— lack of energy
— night sweats
— weight gain
— vaginal dryness
— osteoporosis

Menopause and the Thyroid

Thyroid imbalance can produce many symptoms similar to perimenopause such as weight gain, mood swings, dry skin and low libido. Plus, underlying thyroid imbalances often accelerate during menopause. So please get your thyroid levels checked.

— mood swings
— joint pain
— irritability
— headaches
— decreased libido
— ageing skin and hair
— depression
— anxiety
— irritability
— poor memory
— belly fat
— hair loss
— loss of confidence
— dizzy spells
— hair growth on face
— painful intercourse
— panic attacks
— weird dreams
— fatigue

What Causes these Symptoms?

You guessed it… your hormones. It's the ups and downs and overall decline in hormones that can cause perimenopausal problems. For example, with oestrogen declining more gradually than progesterone, this can leave us oestrogen dominant at times – something we know contributes to hot flushes. Hormones are also exacerbated by stress, weight gain and poor dietary choices.

Declining testosterone can leave us feeling like we'd rather watch paint dry than have sexual relations of any sort, as well as affecting muscle mass and strength, causing skin to thin and become dry.

So What Can we Do?

You may wish to go straight on to hormone replacement therapy (HRT) or bioidentical hormone replacement therapy (BHRT), but to me that's simply another sticking plaster. Your body starts to rely on the adrenal glands to produce the sex hormones once your ovaries hand over the baton, so by supporting this gland through diet and lifestyle changes, we can make the transition smoother.

If you truly commit to this programme, it will tell us one of two things: either you are able to soothe and correct your symptoms and imbalances, or you need further assessments. If it is the latter, by committing and completing the programme you will have set up the environment to better respond to treatment like HRT. *See* Pillar Two: Balance (pages 64–67) and Pillar Six: Restore (pages 78–81).

The menopause is not a disease or a medical condition. Menopause signifies a major transition in a woman's life

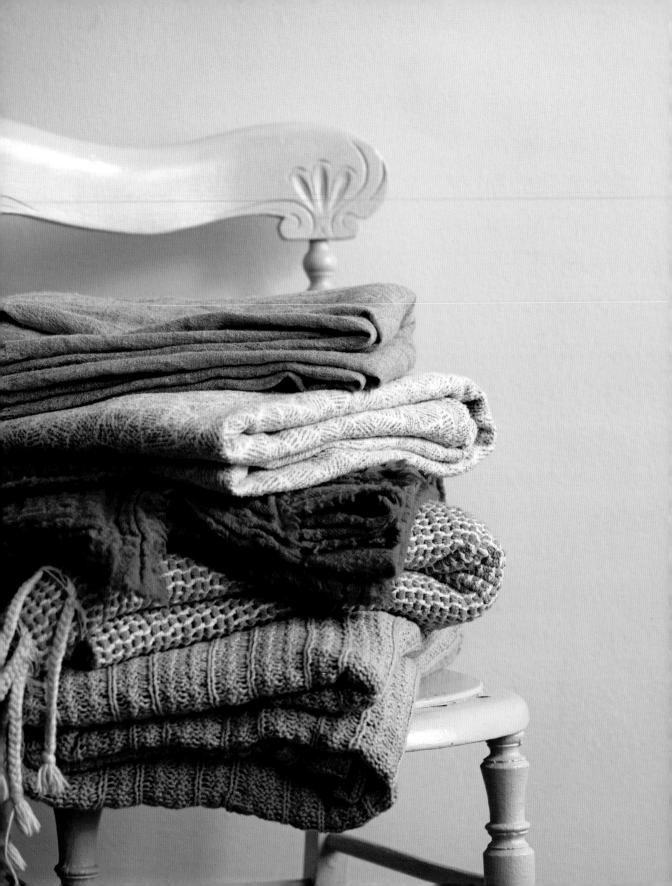

the six pillars of balance

Which Pillars Should You Lean On?

I'm now going to introduce you to the Six Pillars around which my Balance Plan is based. Read through them all, because they will all be relevant to you – our hormones work in synergy, after all. What you will find, however, is some Pillars jump out as more important to you. It may be that your diet is lacking, so Nourish is the Pillar that needs your immediate attention. Or, perhaps, you're so busy, overworked and stressed that Nurture and Restore are where you'll need to focus most. As you read through, I'm sure there will be some lightbulb moments where you think 'Yes! I really need to make this change.'

This section is all important and each Pillar complements the others, so take your time and take it all in. There's a lot covered here, but there's no need to feel overwhelmed. Although the aim of the programme is to incorporate each Pillar into your daily life, I'm looking for progress, not perfection.

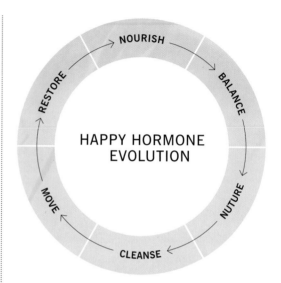

'Me time' is not a luxury, it's a necessity. Remember to take a moment to stop and breathe.

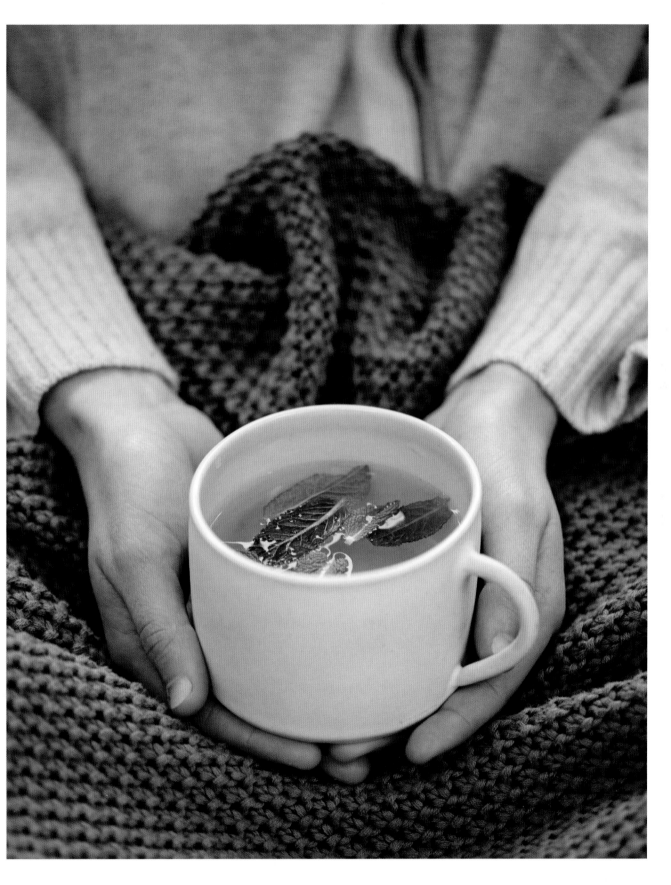

Nourish

Optimally functioning hormones need a steady stream of nutrients in order to work efficiently, so we need to change the way we think about food. The good news is that a few easy tweaks to our diet can make a huge difference to our hormonal balance, virtually straight away.

We tend to eat on the go, distracted by life and not thinking about what we are eating. But food is information and that information is passed to your genes, cells, hormones and metabolism. Optimal nutrition is not just about warding off illness and disease; it is about nourishing the body for an abundance of vitality and a positive and balanced outlook.

Nourish is perhaps the overall aim of the Balance Plan – with its four-week meal plan and delicious recipes to follow. You can read the what-to-eat specifics in more detail from page 82; what follows here are my highlights. But it's not just about what you eat. We are going to change the way you think about food with some easy steps: food is there to be enjoyed, so don't make it a daily battle.

House Rules:

Eat Whole Food, Not Processed Junk Food

Processed foods are devoid of nutrients. Dump the junk and always shop in the outer perimeters of the supermarket for nutrient-dense whole foods. Only enter the middle, the shop's very own Bermuda triangle, to get things like olive oil, nuts and seeds, nut butters, herbal teas and essentials, like loo paper. But wear blinkers as there are shiny packages there to tempt you.

Eat the Right Carbs, Not No Carbs

I know, gasp, carbs? Yes the right carbohydrates are extremely beneficial to us. These are brown and fibrous wholegrains and vegetables, and are what we call slow-release or complex carbohydrates. They're nutrient packed and contain the all-important fibre we need for healthy elimination. Avoid white carbs that are refined – white bread, pasta, white rice, cakes, biscuits, pastries – and no added sugar or artificial sweeteners (*see* page 92).

Eat Good Fats Daily

Fat does not make you fat, sugar does. Eating the right fats in the right amounts builds hormones, reduces inflammation and keeps our cells and skin supple (*see* page 93).

Eat a Rainbow of Vegetables

Fill your plate with different-coloured vegetables – it's the pigments in them that indicate the different nutrients, so the wider the variety of colours, the more vitamins and minerals you'll pack in. Aim for five to ten portions a day. (A portion is the size of your fist, about 80g/3oz.)

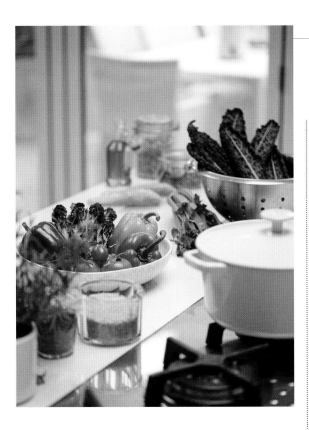

Eat Whole Fruit Only, No Fruit Juice

Enjoy one to two pieces of fruit a day, skin, core and all where possible, as whole fruit – not juice – brings with it both fibre and nutrients. Although dried fruit tastes good and contains fibre and nutrients, it is a concentrated form of fruit sugar and can spike your blood-sugar levels, so best limit it.

Add in Detox Warriors Every Day

Instead of going on a cleanse or detox you are going to love your liver and hormones daily by bringing in detoxing foods like cruciferous and dark green leafy vegetables into your daily diet. Your detox warriors will help clear those spent hormones, keep the liver functioning optimally as it builds new

Chase the nutritional rainbow and fill your kitchen with fresh, colourful fruit and vegetables, good fats and healthy protein. Crowd out the junk food.

hormones and help keep waste products moving out as they should.

Feed Your Eco-warriors

You need to give the good guys in your gut the right foods to flourish and maintain the microbiota diversity you need for digestion, immunity and hormone balance. Eat fermented foods, prebiotics and loads of fibre.

Good Quality Protein Daily

Aim for organic and grass-fed protein when you can – I would rather you ate less of the good stuff than loads of animal produce that is full of hormones and antibiotics and beans and pulses slathered in pesticides and insecticides. Have a good mix of both plant and animal based protein (*also see* page 92 for protein choices).

Reduce Inflammation

Chronic inflammation is not doing your hormonal harmony any favours. In the four-week plan, we are going to aim to reduce inflammation with an array of vegetables and the anti-inflammatory superheroes turmeric and ginger.

Have a Green Smoothie a Day

Green smoothies are high in fibre, detox warriors and magnesium as well as other nutrients. They are like a multivitamin in a glass. Try the smoothie recipes on pages 108–110 and see which one you like the best.

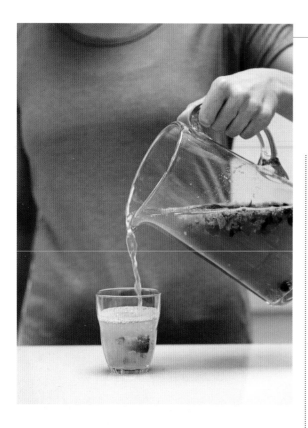

Create a fantastically healthy alternative to fizzy drinks by infusing sparkling water with your favourite fruits and vegetables. For a sparkling twist that is packed full of antioxidants, see my Berry & Mint Fizz recipe on page 111.

Go Organic as Much as Your Budget Allows

This reduces toxic burden and helps with hormonal balance as exposure to xenoestrogens, antibiotics and hormones in animal products, chemicals in fertilizers, pesticides and herbicides all act as a showstopper for our Sassy Six (and the planet).

Say No to Gluten…

We're not just jumping on the 'gluten-free' craze here. There is a lot of research showing that gluten can be extremely inflammatory in the gut and cause bloating and discomfort. Your four-week meal plan is naturally gluten-free (*see* pages 98–105), but after that you may want to reintroduce gluten in small amounts (*see* page 97).

… and Dairy

Again, another big one. We are working to balance your hormones, and unfortunately dairy comes with a host of animal hormones, including oestrogen, and if non organic, it's filled with chemicals and antibiotics. As with gluten, your meal plan (*see* pages 98–105) is dairy-free, but after the four-week meal plan you may want to reintroduce dairy in small amounts (*see* page 97 for how to do this).

Stay Hydrated

Use pure filtered water and herbal teas to keep hydrated throughout the day. Being dehydrated can affect your concentration, mood, digestion, hair, skin and energy levels, not to mention the strain it puts on the body as we need to be well hydrated to function optimally. If you struggle drinking plain water, try infusing it with some mint and fruit for natural, sugar-free flavour.

Avoid Caffeine, Alcohol and Stimulants

Tricky if you rely on coffee to get through the day and wine to unwind, but trust me you don't need them. Your hormones and energy levels will benefit. If you rely on these, wean yourself off slowly.

Mindful Eating Practice

Mindfulness is about being 'in the moment', free from distraction. Digestion starts from the moment you put a piece of food in your mouth, so take time to chew it properly and you'll kick-start the all-important digestive process. Take time over your meals and you'll allow your digestion time to do what it needs to do – and your satiety cues to switch on when you've had enough, too.

The easiest way to practise mindful eating, even if it's just a snack, is to really use your senses. How does the food look, how does it taste, smell, feel in your mouth? Savour whatever you're eating. Connect with it. Mastering the art of eating intelligently is far more important than counting calories. Ask yourself these questions:
— do I multitask when I eat?
— do I eat slowly, chewing each bite properly?
— do I recognize when I slip into mindless zoned-out eating?
— do I stop eating when I am full?

Concentrate, Connect, Nourish

We all tend to rush around from one task to the next, eating at our desks while still typing that email reply, eating while cleaning up or walking to the car, eating in front of the TV, engrossed in the show but distracted from our food. This might seem like multitasking at its best, but at what cost to your hormonal balance? If you eat while you are stressed, blood is diverted away from the digestive track, making digestion harder and causing food to sit there for longer and ferment, leading to bloating and cramping. Being distracted and eating fast also means you eat mindlessly and a lot more than you actually need.

Practise the Attitude of Food Gratitude

Give thanks before you eat. This can mean anything to you, whatever you believe in. Just take a moment to be grateful for the meal you are about to eat and acknowledge the privilege of being able to enjoy this nourishing food.

Take 30

Take time to eat your meal: honestly there isn't a lion chasing you and if there was, would you really still try to finish your lunch? You deserve a 30-minute break to eat in peace. This will allow you to eat consciously and slowly, to really tune into your hunger and satiety signals, giving yourself plenty of time for your brain to get the message that you are in fact full so that you avoid overeating.

No Distractions

I know it's not always possible, but try to have no distractions, other than a friendly conversation with your partner or friends. I love connecting with family at dinner time and sharing the day's events: TV off, no other disturbances. Dining for one? Play some classical music; breathe; connect with your food.

Balance

The foundations of balanced hormones are balanced blood-sugar levels. This stabilizes our insulin, cortisol, androgens and SHBG, leading to better moods, easier sleep, reduced PMS and less of that dreaded, self-perpetuating tummy fat. The other key part of this Pillar is the gut. I always say a poo a day keeps the doctor away, but there is more to it than just having a daily bowel movement. There is a strong correlation between gut health and hormonal health.

The 80/20 rule

I stick to healthy eating 80 per cent of the time and allow for a few indulgences in the remaining 20 per cent. For me, this 20 per cent still centres around natural sugars. At first, my 20 per cent included cakes and anything sweet, but over time my taste buds changed and I wanted different foods.

After the four-week meal plan, follow the Six Pillars 80 per cent of the time, and for the remaining 20 per cent, let your hair down and go with the flow. You will be amazed how good you will feel. Remember, it's about consistency above perfection.

12 Steps to Jumping off the Blood-sugar Roller-coaster

1. Get a Good Night's Rest
Disrupted sleep and circadian rhythms (sleep-wake cycles) lead to elevated glucose and insulin levels.

2. Plan Ahead
How many times have you grabbed a chocolate bar, sandwich or packet of sweets on the run? Avoid temptation and making 'sugary' decisions by planning ahead.

3. Eat Regularly
If you skip meals or leave many hours between them, blood-sugar levels can dip so low they crash. Make time for three evenly spaced main meals a day and avoid mindless snacking in between.

4. Make Breakfast a Priority
Have a good, protein-rich breakfast within an hour of rising to start the morning well, boost your mental energy and set your hormone pattern for the day.

5. Add Good-quality Protein to Every Meal or Snack
Protein keeps you feeling fuller for longer and slows the release of sugar from carbohydrate foods, which means fewer blood-sugar spikes and dips (*see* page 92).

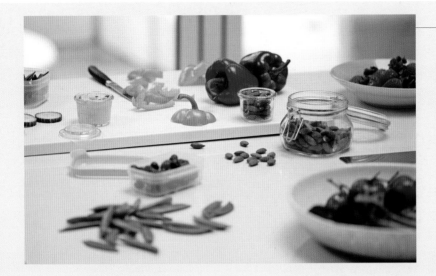

By enjoying the 80/20 rule and jumping off the blood-sugar roller-coaster, you'll be able to find consistency rather than perfection. Embrace your new, balanced lifestyle.

6. Favour those Healthy Fats

Like protein, healthy fats help to slow the release of sugar from carbohydrate foods and keep you feeling fuller for longer.

7. Avoid Sugar and Artificial Sweeteners

Sugar is sugar, whether it's in refined or raw form. Read the ingredients labels and watch for sugar's many guises (syrups and names ending in –ose, like sucrose or dextrose). Artificial sweeteners such as aspartame, saccharin and sucralose are chemicals, not food, and can contribute to insulin resistance and perpetuate a sweet tooth.

8. Avoid Anything White or Fluffy

Our definition of what sugar is needs to be expanded; it is not just the white crystallized stuff. White bread, pastry, pasta and fluffy processed high-GI carbs all convert into sugar within minutes of being eaten.

9. Add Some Cinnamon to Meals

This is one of my secret weapons that I hope you will love. Cinnamon can improve insulin sensitivity and help with blood-sugar balance. Plus it's naturally sweet in taste and can help keep those pesky cravings at bay. Sprinkle a teaspoon of ground cinnamon on breakfast or make a cinnamon tea.

10. Get Moving

Exercise improves your energy, metabolism, insulin balance and self-esteem.

11. Avoid Stimulants

Alcohol and caffeine can stimulate your adrenal glands and increase your cortisol levels. Remember to wean yourself off slowly.

12. Manage Stress

Cortisol can raise blood-sugar levels and generally unbalance hormones.

Gut Health

Keeping your bowels healthy and moving on a daily basis can be one of the most important steps you take towards optimal health, vitality and balanced hormones. Let's troubleshoot a few common gut issues.

Constipation

If you are constipated you are not eliminating toxins and spent hormones and they can be reabsorbed. How much water have you been drinking? When you drink a lot of caffeine, you can get blocked up when you stop using coffee as a laxative. Try munching on loads of veggies – the fibre will help fluff out stools.

You Bloat, You Burp, You Fart, You Blush

If you are very gassy after meals or you feel a burning sensation in your stomach when you eat and the food just sits there for ages causing reflux, bad breath and stomach upsets it could be down to hypochlorhydria, or low stomach acid. You are not able to break your food down properly and therefore not able to absorb such vital nutrients as B12, iron and calcium; this can lead to inflammation and infections of the intestines.

Food Intolerances

Do certain foods leave you feeling terrible after meals? Bloated? Constipated or with loose stools? The Balance Plan removes wheat, gluten and dairy, which are common culprits.

Eight Principles for Better Digestion

While there's no one diet that suits everyone all of the time, these eight, easy principles can guide everyone to healthier digestion.

1. Colour and Freshness

If your food looks pale, drab and boring, then that is probably the best way to describe its nutritional content. The more naturally colourful a food is, the higher its nutritional content. Not only richer in minerals and vitamins, the colours of a plant are caused by powerful plant compounds called phytonutrients, which have been shown to have powerful healing, antioxidant and anti-inflammatory properties.

2. Eco-warriors

We need a favourable balance of healthy versus unhealthy bacteria in our guts. Achieve it with a varied, natural diet, including plenty of pre- and probiotic foods. Prebiotics are fibre-rich foods that 'fertilize' our gut bacteria. They include onions, leeks, garlic, pulses, bananas, Jerusalem artichokes, asparagus, nuts and seeds, cabbage, chicory root and apple. Probiotic foods are fermented and contribute to the healthy bacteria in our guts. They include sauerkraut, kefir, tempeh, kimchi, miso, natto, kombucha and fermented vegetables.

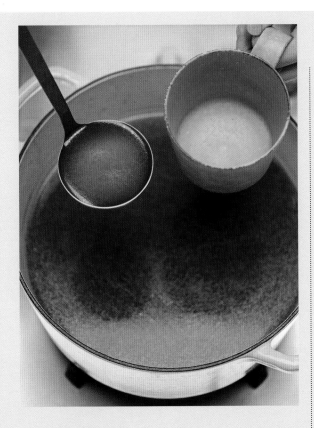

3. Bone Broth (*shown above*)

Filled with amino acids and nutrients, simple bone broth is a gut-reparative food. It's also great for supporting immune system health, as well as repairing joints and connective tissue. Just follow my Chicken Stock recipe on page 166 using your preferred bones of choice.

4. Variety

Variety is the spice of life, but it's also the foundation of good nutrition. Dairy and wheat are the most commonly overeaten foods and many people find them problematic. Don't get stuck in a 'same food' rut. Mix it up. Be adventurous. Try new foods and spices.

5. Fibre

Vegetables, wholegrains and fruit are all high in fibre which helps bulk out the stool, and feed our eco-warriors. Brown, fibrous whole foods and whole grains have much more to offer than their over-processed counterparts. Lightly cooked or raw vegetables and fruit like apple, and berries are the basis of a healthy diet.

6. Water

Water is essential for digestion and good bowel function, softening foods and washing away waste products. Avoid drinking too much during a meal as this may dilute digestive enzymes and impede efficient digestion. Caffeinated beverages do not count – only water truly hydrates, cleans and detoxifies.

7. Chew and relax

Remember your mindful eating practice? Chewing is a big part as it triggers the release of digestive enzymes in the mouth and this, in turn, triggers all the other digestive processes further down the chain. Eating while stressed and on the run can further hinder digestion and throw it out of balance. If you want to digest your food properly, absorb the nutrients and produce less uncomfortable gas, get chewing in a relaxed environment.

8. Exercise

Getting regular moderate exercise is also extremely beneficial to your digestive function and can help alleviate the constipation. I find yoga works wonders for my digestion!

Nurture

You don't have to sit and 'Om' for hours a day to get the benefit of meditation. Even five minutes of restorative breathing can have a positive impact.

This Pillar is about caring for the adrenals and thyroid – our stress and master metabolism glands. Remember that the message of stress overrides any other message in the body. In this Pillar, we aim to reduce the stress response, and to supply the body with the nutrients it needs to support and optimize your day-to-day life. To successfully combat stress and find balance, we need to activate the body's natural relaxation response.

Learn 4/7 Breathing

Adjust your posture to relax your shoulders, and sit comfortably. Keep one hand on your chest and the other on your abdomen. Take a deep breath in for a count of four, expanding your chest and right down into your belly, feeling it expand last. Pause and then breathe out for a count of seven, contracting your belly first, and then chest, as the air leaves your body. Repeat this ten times. Do this every morning and every evening. It's also a handy trick to practise any time you feel anxious, for example if you are stressed at work. Try it if you have difficulty sleeping or you wake in the middle of the night or early morning with an active brain.

The Breath of Life

Breathing is such a natural reflex we tend not to think about how we do it. But breathing is not just about keeping you alive, it can have a profound effect on your nervous system, too. How do you breathe?

Take a moment to place one hand on your chest and the other on your belly, and just breathe as you normally would. Which hand rises more, the one on the chest or the one on the belly? We tend to do a lot of chest breathing, taking short sharp breaths as we try to navigate our way through a stressful day. Breathing relies on our diaphragm, abdomen and intercostal muscles. Deep belly breathing helps turn down the sympathetic nervous system and activates the parasympathetic nervous system. It brings about a sense of calm, reason and presence. It's an easy technique that you can practise daily to relieve muscle tension and anxiety, and nurture those adrenal glands.

Practise Meditation

Mindfulness and meditation teach you to pay attention to the present moment with openness and acceptance. They help improve focus and concentration, create a space for creativeness and increase our ability to withstand stress. Read more about different techniques in Pillar Six: Restore (*see* pages 78–81).

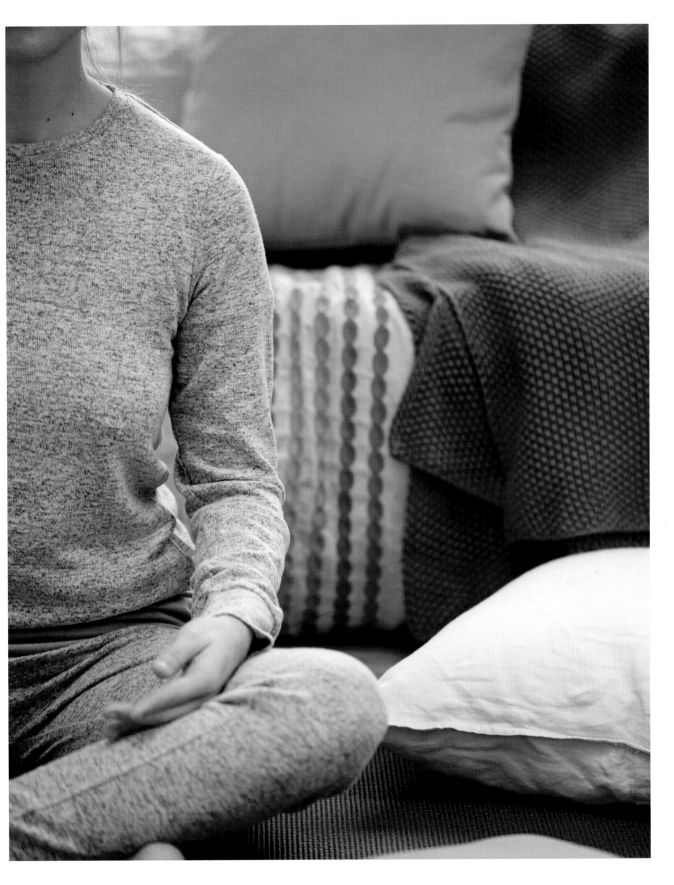

Prioritise Sleep

Sleep is vital for all bodily functions. We need to prioritise good, restorative sleep to nurture our adrenal glands and reduce stress. For proper adrenal rehab we need to start putting a curfew on laptops, computers, tablets and phones. Turn them off a few hours before bed and definitely keep them out of the bedroom. We need a break from that hormone-disrupting blue light (and stress-arousing stimulus) to reset our circadian rhythms and rebalance our cortisol and melatonin levels.

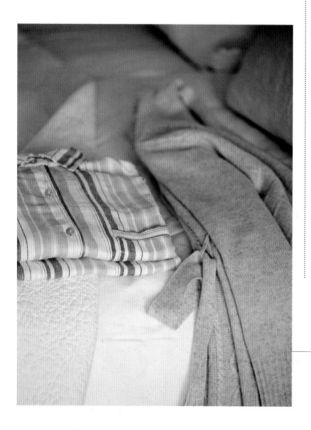

Laugh More

I love chatting about this with clients. When was the last time you just sat and laughed? Laughter is food for the soul and we need to do more of it. Watch a funny movie, go see a stand-up comedy show, read a hilarious book that makes you laugh out loud, spend time with your wittiest friends. Fill your life with more joy.

Change Your Response to Stress

Easier said than done, I know, but it's easy to make a mountain out of a molehill. Have you ever flown off the handle then a few days later thought, 'What on earth was I bothered about?' As you've learned by now, the body doesn't differentiate between real threat and chronic stress, it's all damaging to your hormone balance. If you have a lot of issues to work through, it's well worth speaking to a therapist.

The next time you're faced with a stressful situation and you can feel the anger rising in you, I want you to stop and take a step back. Try the breathing exercise on page 68. Feel better? Yes, that demanding email from your boss needs to be answered, but not at a cost to your health and your Sassy Six. So reply from a

Need more energy in the day? Go to bed early and enjoy more rest. Sleep is an unsung hero and we need to pay more attention to it.

place of calm, then file the email and go about your day. This new approach may take some getting used to, but commit to the process.

Be More Active

When our adrenals are working in overdrive we can feel exhausted, and the last thing we want to do is exercise. But adaptive exercises, like going for a brisk walk outside and filling your lungs with fresh air, can be just what you need to re-energise. Yoga or Pilates, which incorporate deep breathing work, can be extremely restorative, while working on stability and core muscles. Another exercise that doesn't require a lot of exertion if you are feeling depleted is a barre class, or you could even try a mini trampoline rebounder and start with five to ten minutes' jumping, twice a day. You can add in some light weights and body resistance training, like squats and lunges, to increase muscle mass, and therefore increase energy. Getting regular moderate exercise is also extremely beneficial to the thyroid and will help alleviate the constipation that often comes with hypothyroidism. Exercise stimulates thyroid gland secretion and increases tissue sensitivity to the thyroid hormone. I know all too well that having fatigue from an under-functioning thyroid is debilitating, so start small, get quality movement and don't rush – it's not a competition. For more ideas, *see* Pillar Five: Move, on pages 76–77 – but don't neglect this vital element. Get active.

Nurture Your Thyroid

The thyroid needs the following nutrients for optimal functioning. Make sure you're getting a good selection on a regular basis:
— iodine – in fish, eggs and seaweed
— zinc – in meat, shellfish, whole grains and some nuts
— vitamin E – in olive oil, nuts and seeds
— vitamin A – in eggs, oily fish, yellow and orange vegetables
— vitamin B2 (riboflavin) – in eggs and rice
— vitamin B3 (niacin) – in meat, fish, eggs and avocado
— vitamin B6 (pyridoxine) – in poultry, fish, whole grains, vegetables and pulses
— vitamin C – in peppers, broccoli and berries
— selenium – in Brazil nuts, fish, meat and eggs
— vitamin D – sunlight is our main source, but it's available in small amounts in oily fish, egg yolks, liver and mushrooms

When was the last time you just sat and laughed? Laughter is food for the soul and we need to do more of it

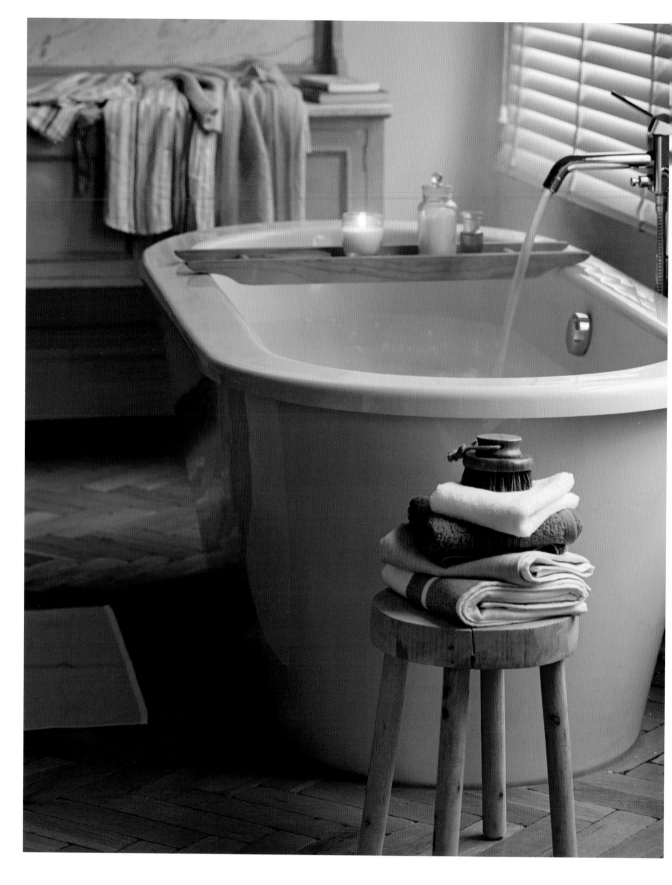

Cleanse

We live in a more toxic world than ever before, being constantly bombarded by harmful chemicals on a daily basis. The scary thing is we aren't always aware of where those toxins are hiding as they are circulating in our environment. Some are more obvious than others but they can be found in everything from our food, water, household and skincare products, to the soil and the air we breathe. To make matters worse, many of the chemicals modern life exposes us to are hormone disruptors, some are even thought to cause some cancers.

Yes, some people argue that there is no connection between environmental toxins and our hormones. But I call BS on that. I've read enough research on the links to be convinced. So this Pillar is about cleaning up our acts. Our bodies detoxify daily, cleaning out waste materials and pollutants to maintain our cellular health. But there are plenty of foods we can add in to support this process – as well as lots we can do to cleanse our immediate environment.

We are what we eat, drink, breathe, touch, absorb and can't eliminate. With that in mind, Cleanse is an extremely important Pillar.

Cleanse Your Body

Start Your Day with a Cup of Warm Water and Lemon Juice

On waking, have a cup of warm water with lemon juice. This will wake your digestion slowly and aid detoxification. I use a straw to protect my teeth from the acidity. You can add anti-inflammatory turmeric and soothing ginger, if you like.

Filter Your Water

Drink only filtered water where you can. I have a water filter attached to my drinking-water supply at home. It was a big investment, but I feel better drinking the water. You can get countertop water filters as well, of course, but those at the cheaper end won't remove substances such as synthetic oestrogen. Use a glass water jug or ensure that it's BPA free.

Buy Food Unwrapped

Choose whole foods with as little packaging as possible to reduce your exposure to chemicals and toxins found in plastics and canned products. Don't wrap food in clingfilm.

Have Detox Warriors Daily

Chase the rainbow and spice up your life with our Detox Warriors (*see* page 61 and 92) – foods that help your body to cleanse itself.

Ensure that you are getting a good mix. Have a side of greens with most meals.

Eat Some Ground Flaxseeds Every Day

Have a couple of tablespoons of ground flaxseeds (linseeds) a day. This will help boost fibre and good fats, and a special little compound called lignans in flaxseeds can help balance our hormones. Have them in smoothies, on porridge or sprinkled over salad and vegetables.

Spice up Your Life

As well as adding flavour to food, herbs and spices contain a vast array of phytonutrients, which help support the liver. I love turmeric, ginger, parsley, rosemary, coriander and garlic.

Get Sweaty

Get your trainers on and get moving, because sweat plays a crucial role in your body's natural detox function and helps clear out a range of toxins, from those pesky persistent organic pollutants (POPs) and BPA to heavy metals (along with that alcohol you drank last night!). Spending time in a sauna counts, too; the most benefit is seen from infrared saunas. Remember to rehydrate to replace the water lost.

Try an Epsom Salt Bath

Have a detoxifying bath in Epsom salts, otherwise known as magnesium sulphate, which is easily absorbed through our skin. Not only is an Epsom salt bath blissfully relaxing, it aids in the elimination of toxins and waste by stimulating your lymph system and encouraging increased oxygen and blood flow. Draw a hot bath, add one to three cups of salts and soak in it for up to half an hour. Do this a couple of times a month. You can add relaxing lavender oil for an extra treat.

Dry-brush it Off

This simple detoxifying technique only takes five minutes a day, exfoliates dead skin, enhances your circulation and stimulates the lymphatic system. You need a natural bristle brush with a long handle so you can reach all

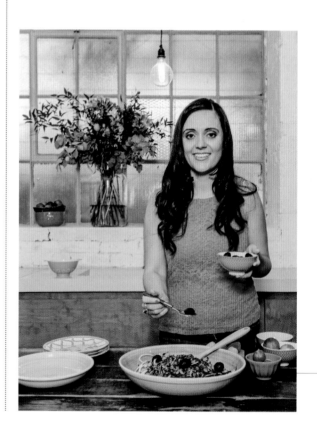

areas of your body. Do this naked just before a shower – I find mornings are best. Start at your feet and, using gentle, long sweeping motions or circular movements, brush towards your heart (take care as you brush over more sensitive areas like breasts).

Cleanse Your Environment

Don't do Plastic
Avoid drinking from plastic water bottles and travel mugs as much as possible, and do not wash plastic food or beverage containers under high heat. Do not heat plastic in the micowave.

Be a Storage Guru
Use glass, stainless steel or ceramic containers instead of plastic containers for heating and storing hot food. Don't put any plastic containers into the microwave.

Look for BPA-free Products
Avoid using vinyl clingfilm and food cans that are lined with BPA, which can leach into the food.

Eat Organic
Invest in organic produce whenever possible, and minimize consumption of high-mercury fish, such as fresh tuna, marlin or swordfish.

What's on the end of your fork matters. The more naturally colourful a food is, the higher its nutritional content.

Keep Things Pest Free
Avoid using pesticides/herbicides in the home and garden.

Manage Your Cycle Ethically
Use organic, unbleached cotton sanitary products that are chemical free, ethical, environmental and animal-friendly and biodegradable. Try a reusable Moon Cup – a soft, medical-grade silicone menstrual cup that is safe and eco-friendly.

Be a Smart Label Reader
Avoid cosmetics, deodorants, anti-bacterial soap, shampoo, toothpaste, hair care and sun care products, and other beauty products containing parabens and phthalates. Don't buy anything that says 'fragranced' or 'perfumed'. The skin is our largest organ and will absorb whatever you put on it.

Get Fresh
Air fresheners and scented candles are loaded with chemicals and, though they smell good, they are not doing your hormones any favours. Look for organic, non-petrochemical candles, or use essential oils to freshen the room.

Clean Green
Get rid of the toxin-laden cleaning products in your house. Choose natural, chemical-free products or try using vinegar, water and lemon juice, and baking soda like our grannies did.

Move

Exercise is essential not only for our overall fitness and health, but for our hormonal health, too. Too little won't work, but too much can be a stress on the body and wipe out some of the benefits, so it pays to spend a little time figuring out what works best for you. I'm not a personal trainer; this is basic advice and, hopefully, inspiration.

There are so many benefits to exercising and it plays a role in each of the other Pillars. We know it can help relieve stress and reduce cortisol levels, make our cells more sensitive to thyroid hormones and insulin, help with elimination and detoxification, and increase energy. If done correctly it can have a massive benefit on your Sassy Six. Need more convincing? Moving more...

— supports bone health
— increases lung capacity
— improves the circulation of oxygen, getting those all-important nutrients around the body
— helps to alleviate low mood by stimulating endorphins
— improves mental clarity, as it stimulates your brain
— strengthens the heart
— improves blood and lymphatic flow
— builds muscle
— helps burn fat
— boosts confidence and self-esteem
— alleviates back pain
— promotes better sleep

What's Your Excuse?

Modern life can be a real barrier to exercise. We've all become more sedentary and technology driven, but it comes at a cost to our health. Maybe you drive a car or take public transport, reducing the amount of walking you do (the simplest form of exercise). Perhaps you're exhausted from working long hours and just don't feel like working out. Or you have a mental struggle with exercise, and find it really hard to get going. I used to loathe exercise, and then I started exercising obsessively to punish myself – it was a long battle. These days I work out at least three times a week, for 30 minutes to an hour, and get some form of movement in every day, even if it's just a 10 minute walk. You should aim for the same. Try saying this affirmation every time you exercise: 'I work out because I love my body'.

Find Your Fitness

Moderate exercise reduces cortisol levels and reaps all the benefits listed. But exercising excessively can disrupt your hormones and cause adrenal insufficiency. This creates too much free-radical formation, which can also speed up the ageing processes considerably and impair the immune system.

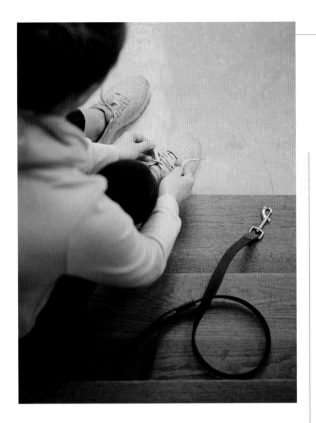

Sitting is the new smoking and, as most of us work long hours in sedentary jobs, it's important you find time to get moving. This is a nutritionist's order – it's essential for your hormones and overall health.

Movement should energize you and not exhaust you. Start small and build up, but commit to daily movement. It doesn't always need to be a 'trainers, Lycra and sweat band' kind of event; gentle movement counts too. Put a movement appointment in your diary as a non-negotiable appointment with yourself.

Some More Ways to Get Moving

— meet friends for walks rather than coffee and cake dates
— take the stairs, not the lift
— get off the bus a stop early, or walk the whole way
— take the dog for more walks (no dog? Borrow one!)
— get a pedometer or activity tracker, or download an app to your smartphone to monitor movement and motivate yourself
— choose active hobbies – gardening, DIY, visiting museums and galleries
— get the kids off the sofa and away from video games – go for a family stroll or kick-about in the park
— take up dance class or dance in the living room

We are all biochemically individual. You need to find what works for you, what you enjoy and what fits in with your lifestyle.

We mentioned a few ideas already in Pillar Four: Nurture (*see* pages 68–71). What about a dance class like Zumba or high-intensity interval training (HIIT)? – a short and sweet way of working out that has lots of positive research to support its health and fitness benefits. Hate going to the gym? Going for a gentle jog – there are plenty of books, apps and podcasts that can help you get you from couch to 5km in a few weeks. You could a join a local walking group, cycling club or take a yoga or dance class.

Restore

As women, we are professional plate-spinners. Day in, day out, we keep those plates spinning – work, family, friends, pets, exercise, cooking, socializing – without dropping any of them. But sooner or later something's going to get smashed if we don't have the resources to enable us to do all this multitasking.

In Pillar Six, we work on getting better sleep, which is when repair and healing happens. We create 'me time', we start a daily meditation practice to stimulate the parasympathetic nervous system (where digestion and hormones work). We learn how to practise an attitude of gratitude that will help us create the inner peace that is so important for stress reduction, improved mood and good digestion, all of which contribute to hormonal balance.

When I talk about this to the ladies in my clinic or workshop I am often met with 'What me time?' or 'I'd feel too guilty if I did that', or, my personal favourite: 'Who will do all the housework and get the kids ready if I am sat on my backside saying "Om"?'. But making time for this Pillar is essential. We want to ensure that your mental, emotional and spiritual needs are being met.

Consider these questions for a moment:
— When was the last time you fully relaxed?
— How did you feel while you were doing it?
— How did you feel after you finished?
— Did the world keep turning while you were relaxing?
— Was everybody still ok?

You've heard the saying 'You can't pour from an empty cup'. We need to fill your cup. Your reserve tank needs to be bursting so that you can feel revitalized and rejuvenated. The key is to find simple daily things that help the restorative process, as well as more significant steps like massage or holidays. It's easy to turn to things like TV, alcohol, snacks or even our smartphones when we think we need to de-stress. This Pillar is about using our downtime more productively, restoring our bodies and minds with techniques scientifically proven to promote healing and renewal, and triggering lasting improvements to health and hormones.

Get a Good Night's Sleep
We have already discussed the importance of a good night's sleep for better hormonal balance, weight, mood, motivation and control over our cravings, but many of us are just not getting it. You should be having a solid eight hours of sleep every night. Consider your past few nights in bed. Are you sleeping enough? Are you sleeping well through the night, waking up refreshed? What are the obstacles or challenges that make it harder for you to sleep? What can you change?

Try These Sleep-better Tips

— Get enough daylight (during the day) to help maintain your circadian rhythms. Walk to work, have lunch outside or go for a stroll in the park.

— Make the bedroom your sanctuary – take out all electronics and create a technology-free zone.

— Ensure your room is pitch black to help stimulate melatonin – get black-out blinds or curtains if you need to, put tape over LED lights and consider wearing an eye mask.

— Don't watch scary or stimulating movies, TV shows or read stimulating books before bed.

— Do your 4/7 breathing (see page 68) before bed.

— Get into a routine. Go to bed at the same time every night and tell yourself it's bed time. Aim to be in bed and asleep most nights between 10 and 10:30pm.

— Sprinkle a couple of drops of lavender essential oil onto your pillow.

— Get a soothing alarm clock to wake you up, like a light alarm clock that mimics the sunrise, or one with birds chirping, or the sound of whales instead of something that scares the hell out of you every morning. You want to wake in a calm state, not straight into fight or flight.

— Don't eat too close to bed time; have your meal at least three to four hours earlier.

— Drink a cup of chamomile or valerian tea one hour before bed.

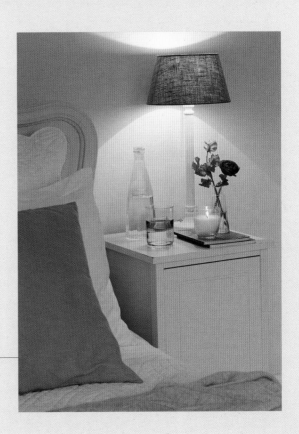

Make your bedroom a calming sanctuary, free from clutter and technology: somewhere to retreat to for a restorative night's sleep.

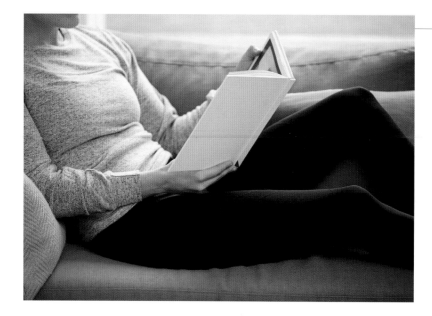

When did you last allow yourself to get lost in a good book or glossy magazine? Prioritize yourself – you have to take care of you before you can take care of everyone else.

Take 'Time Out'

Choose a moment in every day, whether it's ten minutes or one hour, to take time out. You can have a quiet cup of herbal tea, read a magazine, have a long soak in the bath, sing in the shower, do your 4/7 breathing (explained on page 68) or a guided meditation. Whatever you choose, make sure it's time just for you.

Be Social

Arrange a girly lunch or night on the town. Get together with a group of friends who inspire and empower you, and make you laugh out loud. Don't hide away: we are social creatures, so find your tribe and nurture those relationships.

Get Lost

Not literally, but set your mind free on walks in nature, in a funny movie or in a conversation where you are totally present. It helps us shift to being rather than just doing.

Spend Time Visualizing and Saying Positive Affirmations

I love the power of positivity. Start each day by looking at yourself in a mirror and speaking aloud one of the following affirmations (or one you write yourself):

— I can and will make positive choices
— I choose to eat healthy foods
— Each day I am empowered by what I have achieved
— I eat when I am calm and relaxed
— I take time for me every day
— My hormones are balanced and happy
— I am focused on giving my body all it needs
— I love and nurture my amazing body
— I love to move my body daily
— I can do this
— The better I eat, the more I rest, the better I feel
— I am grateful for all the blessings in my life

Meditate

With so many free resources available to help you meditate it has never been easier, and no, you don't have to chant 'Om' if you don't want to! Meditation has been practised by many cultures all over the world for thousands of years, and the proven health benefits include a reduction in pain, anxiety, depression and stress. Because meditation reduces cortisol levels, improved concentration and creativity can result, too. In short, your entire body and mind are affected in a positive way. Meditation is easily done while lying down, sitting or even walking, and as long as you can achieve a calm and positive state of mind there really are no rules. See the box on the right for some of my preferred meditation techniques.

Focus on Gratitude

The act of expressing gratitude has been linked to many improved physical, psychological and social health benefits. Start or end each day by writing down three to five things that you are grateful for in life, big or small. This puts us in the frame of mind of positivity, a focus on all the good we already have and how blessed our lives are. You can be grateful for things that are still coming, for example, I am grateful for my beautifully balanced hormones. Or I am grateful for the me time I will be getting this afternoon. Avoid repeating the same entries, but challenge yourself to allow your awareness and sense of gratitude to flourish.

Treat Yourself

OK, most of us can't fit these in daily, but every so often try to book yourself a massage or a manicure, or take yourself off to the theatre, out for dinner or whatever makes you happy. Book a mini break or a longer holiday if you can. It doesn't have to cost the earth – visit friends or have a staycation – just be sure to stop work, unplug and wind down.

Finding a Meditation Practice that Suits You

I personally like guided meditation and I recommend yoga nidra meditation and also Sophrology, which uses a blend of Eastern and Western philosophies and practices, combining breathing, visualization, gentle movement and relaxation techniques to bring about dynamic relaxation.

If you can't find a class there are all sorts of books, websites and apps that can explain different techniques. Try several until you find something that works for you, even if it's just spending a few moments each morning sitting quietly and listening to the sound of your own breath.

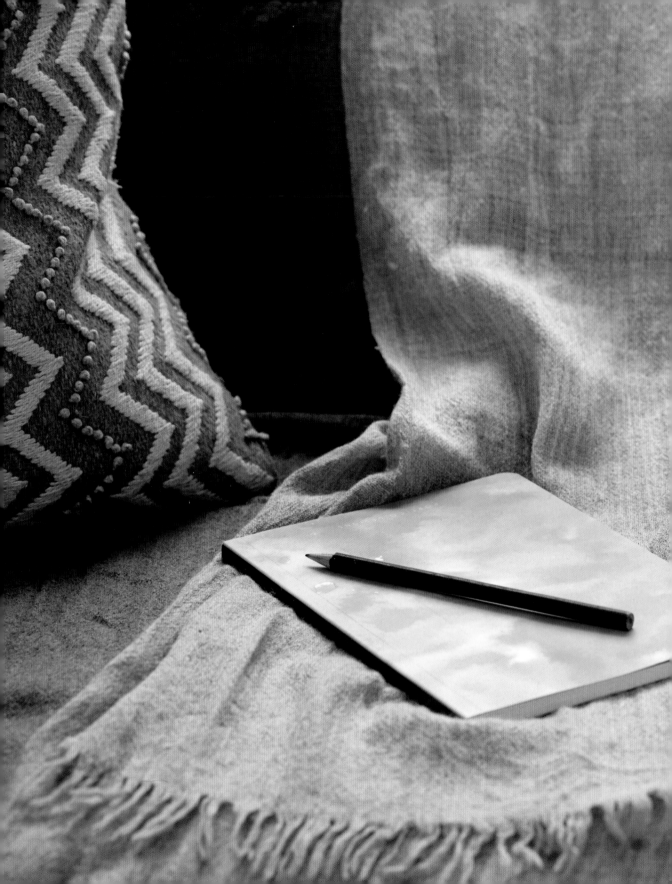

your personal plan

Your Food Diary

So you've done the background reading, you've learned all about your Sassy Six and you've familiarized yourself with the Showstoppers that can unbalance your hormones. You've also got to grips with the Six Pillars that will form your new approach to a balanced, healthy life. It's nearly time to get started on my four-week meal plan, but first let's find out where you're starting from.

It's Time to Play Detective

I'd like you to fill out a food diary for the next one to two weeks. Include every morsel and sip that passes your lips and at what time – you should be leaving four to five hours between meals, interspersed with snacks only if absolutely necessary; you should not be perpetually grazing. But not just that, I also want you to log how you're feeling each day, what digestive or other symptoms you have, how active you were, how stressed you felt, how much 'me time' you had, how you slept – oh and how your bowel movements were. I'd also like you to keep a running cost of how much you think you spend on food and drink each day, especially if you're buying snacks or meals when out and about.

You'll find a blank copy of this two-week food diary on the following pages for you to fill in (or you can photocopy it or copy it out). When you have a week or two's entries, it's time to look for patterns so you can build a picture of your current diet and lifestyle.

Take a red marker and highlight:
— all the sweet foods
— all the white, refined carbs
— any stimulants like coffee, tea, energy drinks, soda pops, alcohol
— any 'diet' or 'sugar-free' products
— any processed junk foods, high in trans or hydrogenated fats
— every time you skipped a meal
— every time you ate on the run
— moods – highlight when you felt stressed, moody, irritable, or had insomnia or were tired
— digestion – if you were bloated, burpy, flatulent, constipated or had diarrhoea

How Much are You Spending?

You may be wondering why I've asked you to note how much money you spend on meals, drinks and snacks each day. This is because people often worry that following a healthy eating plan is expensive and involves lots of costly supplements and superfoods. I want you to realize how much you're currently spending on junk – and how a healthy diet based on natural, whole foods will probably cost you less, not more.

Next, take a green marker and highlight:

— all the vegetables you ate
— all the good-quality protein you ate
  like chicken, eggs, turkey, lamb, fish,
  beans and pulses
— all the times you ate complex carbs
  like brown rice, sweet potatoes, quinoa,
  butternut squash
— all the water, herbal teas or vegetable
  smoothies
— all the good fats you had like nuts
  and seeds, avocado, olive oil, fish
— the days you had three meals a day
— every time you exercised
— all the nights you were in bed before
  midnight and had a good night's rest
— mood – every time you were happy,
  felt satisfied or content
— digestion – every time you had a
  proper stool movement
— me time – every time you were able to
  relax, meditate and do something for you

Next, take a yellow marker and highlight:

— all the fruit you ate
— how many times a day you ate wheat
  or gluten like bread and pasta
— how many times a day you ate dairy
  like milk, cheese, yogurt

The Results

So, now you have a completed food diary that's covered in traffic-light markings! The purpose? To show you how much room for improvement there is – as well as to highlight what you're already doing right.

Any entries that you've marked in red are what you want to phase out during the next four weeks. These sorts of habits aren't going to keep you in balance.

Any entries that you've highlighted green mean you can pat yourself on the back. Let's see if we can turn your whole diary green, going forwards.

Finally, any entries that you've marked yellow aren't necessarily cause for concern, but if having these foods seems also to have caused negative symptoms, you may have a degree of intolerance. Keep a close eye on these possible trigger foods in the future. With regard to fruit, note how many portions you are having: we are aiming for one to two portions a day.

The Next Four Weeks and Beyond

Keep up your diary while you're following the four-week meal plan – and afterwards as you move forwards with your new, balanced life. Keep hold of all your old entries, too. Why? So you can track how you're feeling and how your symptoms are improving or, hopefully, disappearing. Looking back at your old habits and how unwell you sometimes felt can also be great motivation to keep up your new, healthier habits.

Your Food Diary: Week One

Date and Time	Food and Drink	Mood Thoughts and Feelings	Symptoms	Exercise and Movement (Type, Duration and Effort out of 10)
Monday				
Tuesday				
Wednesday				
Thursday				
Friday				
Saturday				
Sunday				

Bowel Movements	Stool Type (*see* Poo Chart on Page 48)	Stress Levels (on a Scale of 1–10)	Me Time	Sleep Time and Quality	Cost of Food and Drink

Your Food Diary: Week Two

Date and Time	Food and Drink	Mood Thoughts and Feelings	Symptoms	Exercise and Movement (Type, Duration and Effort out of 10)
Monday				
Tuesday				
Wednesday				
Thursday				
Friday				
Saturday				
Sunday				

Bowel Movements	Stool Type (*see* Poo Chart on Page 48)	Stress Levels (on a Scale of 1–10)	Me Time	Sleep Time and Quality	Cost of Food and Drink

Monitor Your Progress

Before you begin the plan I'd also like you to jot down some personal data, so you can compare your before and after statistics (for another feel-good boost).

Keep a note of:
— your measurements – chest, waist, hips, upper arm and thigh
— your weight
— your waist-to-hip ratio – which is your waist measurement divided by your hip measurement

It's also a nice idea to ask someone to take before and after photographs of you (or you can take selfies). Wear underwear or slim-fitting sports gear and take full-length snaps from the front, side and back. Take some close-up, make-up free photos of your face, too.

Scared About Making Food Changes?

I know it can be daunting, but if you want to feel better you need to switch things up. And nobody else can do it for you! One definition of insanity is doing the same thing and expecting a different result. It's time to move out of your comfort zone.

Repeat all these measurements and photos after the four weeks – and at any point in the future as you continue with the plan (I like to ask clients to repeat them after two and three months). Seeing your positive results will really spur you on to keep going.

The Balance Plan is not a weight-loss programme per se, it's about bringing your body back into equilibrium. That said, everyone who tries it experiences some noteworthy changes to their body shape and general appearance. It might be the dark circles under your eyes or your complexion that changes, or maybe your water retention or cellulite disappears. It's valuable to record all these measurements and photos, so you can monitor changes of all sorts.

How do You Feel?
Finally, I'd like you to think about how you feel, healthwise, on a daily basis. Next to your measurements, jot down a few sentences and list any ailments, symptoms or moods that are a general feature of your life at the moment. I'm talking things like fatigue, acne, PMS, digestive issues, low mood, aches and pains. It's easy to have a selective memory, so by committing these things to paper, you can better see what changes.

Get to Grips with the Four-week Meal Plan

The purpose of my four-week meal plan is to reset your hormones and get you back on an even keel. All your symptoms may not disappear at the end of the four weeks but they didn't all begin in only four weeks, did they? This is your starting point; if you commit you will notice a big change.

The plan comes with all the recipes you need and they are family friendly. I encourage you to give everything a try, even if the foods are new to you or you don't think you'll like them. You will! I have created the plan with busy women in mind, so your dinners will double up as lunch the next day and you can start to prep your breakfast from the night before too.

What's IN:
— hearty nourishing meals
— phytonutrients through a rainbow of colourful vegetables
— good-quality protein
— fibre
— lots of healthy fats
— whole fruit
— naturally gluten-free whole grains
— beans and pulses
— chocolate (in the form of raw cacao)
— organic (where possible)
— fermented foods
— nuts and seeds
— herbal teas
— healthy snacks
— healthy desserts
— pure water
— vegetable smoothies

What's Limited:
— natural sweeteners like honey and maple syrup
— excessive amounts of fruit
— dried fruit

What's OUT:
— refined sugars and anything with an 'ose' (such as sucrose or dextrose)
— refined carbohydrates – anything white, sweet and fluffy
— alcohol
— dairy
— processed foods
— gluten and wheat
— caffeine
— decaf tea or coffee
— margarine
— cooking with refined vegetable oils
— shop bought dressings and condiments
— artificial sweeteners in any form
— low-fat products
— fruit juice

If you have a lot of stimulants like sugar, caffeine and alcohol, use the week before you start the plan to start weaning yourself off of them. You may have withdrawal symptoms such as headaches or even nausea, so go slow!

Your Ideal Plate

Think back to the last meal you ate. What did your plate look like? Was it full of colourful vegetables? A good source of protein, healthy carbs and good fats?

1. Fill half your plate with non-starchy vegetables like dark green leafy vegetables or salad or asparagus, aubergine, avocado, bamboo shoots, broccoli, cabbage, cauliflower, celery, chicory, courgette, cucumber, endive, fennel, garlic, herbs, kale, leeks, lettuce, mangetout, marrow, okra, pak choi, parsley, peppers, radicchio, radish, rocket, spinach, spring greens, sugar snap peas, swiss chard, tomatoes, watercress, artichokes, kohlrabi, mushrooms and onions. Think of vegetables (and fruit like berries, apples or pears) as your 'Detox Warriors' – packed with phytonutrients that support all your body's detoxification organs and benefit all aspects of our health.

2. On one quarter of your plate, add good-quality protein like fish, chicken, meat, beans and pulses, eggs and soy (natto, miso, tempeh). As a guide, your portion should be roughly the size of your palm. Protein is the basis of all living cells. It's essential for a healthy body and balanced hormones. It helps to build lean muscles, balances hormones and gives our body the tools for tissue repair, cell growth, healthy hair and skin, detoxification and a strong immune system. As a bonus, it helps keep our blood-sugar levels balanced and alleviates some hormone fluctuations as well as being involved in their manufacture.

3. On the other quarter, have your whole grains or complex carbohydrates such as brown rice, quinoa, other gluten-free grains, or startchy veg like sweet potato, beetroot, pumpkin, butternut squash, swede, turnips, new potatoes, beans, legumes and pulses. I recommend not having more than 50–80g at a time. That's around a fist size. (If you are insulin resistant I would limit that further and only have them every second day until you have reset your metabolism and become more insulin sensitive.) Remember, carbohydrates aren't evil. In fact, they're one of the three macronutrients we need in our daily diet. It's simply a matter of eating the right ones.

4. So where's the space for our good fats? Rather than thinking about fats as a separate item of food on your plate, incorporate them as an integral part of a food – for example avocado, nuts and seeds, oily fish, olive oil, chia seeds, coconut oil, ground flaxseeds and bone broth.

Note: If you follow this plate recommendation and you feel that you are still hungry or that it doesn't last you long enough, play around with your protein and complex carb portions – you may need a little more protein and a little less complex carbs. Also check that you have enough good fats.

A Word About Fats

The types of fat we should completely avoid are trans or hydrogenated fats and refined vegetable oils, sometimes (although less often these days) found in ready meals, fast food products, processed foods, processed cakes and biscuits. But you won't be having those on the Balance Plan, so they're super easy to avoid!

What are 'good' fats, exactly? Well they include polyunsaturated essential fatty acids omega-3 and 6. Omega-9 (a monounsaturated fat), although not classified as an essential fatty acid, also has health benefits. Consuming these high-quality fats on a daily basis is recommended for hormonal balance, reducing inflammatory pathways, stabilizing blood-sugar levels, improving insulin sensitivity and minimizing sugar cravings.

Omega-3: found in oily fish (such as salmon, mackerel, sardines, herring and fresh tuna), certain seeds (such as linseeds/flaxseeds and their oils, pumpkin seeds and chia seeds) and walnuts, dark green vegetables, egg yolks and wild or pastured raised meats. Research shows a link between increased menstrual pain, infertility, premature birth and even hot flushes when omega-3 blood concentrations are low, so be sure to include them in your daily diet.

Omega-6: found in nuts (especially almonds), seeds (such as pumpkin and chia seeds) pine nuts and oils (such as sesame oil, sunflower oil, walnut seed oil, evening primrose and borage oil).

Omega-9: found in olives, cold-pressed extra virgin olive oil, avocado (avocados and their oils are nutrient dense and antioxidant rich), hazelnut, pecans, almond butter, macadamia nuts and sunflower seeds, pasture-raised or wild meats.

Saturated fats: found in animal products and certain plant foods, can be included in your diet and have been shown to be beneficial – but just remember that moderation and balance are key. All forms of fats, eaten in excess, will lead to weight gain. Virgin coconut oil is a great example of a healthy saturated fat and is perfect for using in cooking and baking. It's a special kind of fat because it contains metabolism-boosting medium-chain triglycerides, which mean they go straight to the liver to be used for energy, rather than stored as fat. Coconut oil is also anti-inflammatory and anti-bacterial because it is rich in lauric acid and monolaurin but, as with everything, have it in moderation. There's also nothing wrong with a scraping of butter after the four-week meal plan – ideally organic butter from grass-fed cows.

A Little Pre-plan Planning...

Here's where you set yourself up for success, because anything is possible. When it comes to goal setting, think big, then start small. Write out your goals in the present tense, for example, "I eat and nourish my body to have better hormonal health".

Here are a few questions to get you thinking:
— What are you hoping to achieve by following this programme?
— What is most important to you?
— What would you like to achieve for your emotional health?
— What are your ideal physical and exercise health goals?

Then take a step back and set smaller goals to get you to this big goal. For example, if you currently skip breakfast, crave caffeine and shun vegetables:
— I'll have a protein-rich breakfast, no more than one hour after rising
— I'll reduce my coffees by half each week
— I'll have one portion of vegetables with each meal this week, rising to two next week

Make a promise to yourself that you'll work towards these goals, and remember to celebrate the wins, however small (just not with a bottle of bubbly!).

Dump the Junk

If you don't have junk food in the home, then you can't eat it. So take some time to purge your cupboards. If like me, you don't like to waste food, give it to someone else or to a food bank, but do get rid of it. I'm talking about all the processed, refined carbohydrates, sugary sweets and tarts, the crisps, bottled and packet sauces, and the frozen meat products that don't have a lot of meat in them and are quite possibly covered in breadcrumbs. The breakfast cereal that is basically just sugar, the nuts that used to be healthy until they were roasted or coated in chocolate. The massive tin of assorted chocolates that were reduced in price so you bought two. And the fizzy drinks, juices and cordials.

What's Holding You Back?

This is a question I always ask clients and it's worth thinking about before you get started, so you don't lose motivation. Here are some common stumbling blocks, or excuses, that I hear about in clinic:

'I don't have enough time'

Yes, we're all busy, but what is the most important thing in your life? Is it your family? Your friends? Your pets? Your work? Financial freedom? Your health should be first on that list. It's not selfish. If you don't prioritize your own health you cannot be there for everyone else. Get up earlier, batch cook meals, stop being such a people pleaser, say no sometimes. Put yourself first.

'I'm scared to change my habits'

This is a real fear, we hold on so tightly to what we know. Who will you be if you are not eating the foods you are used to eating? How will you go out if you cannot drink as much as you used to? Turn these questions and this self-doubt on its head. Think about how long you've been feeling below par and how much more enriched your life could be if you felt better?

What would you let go of, if you knew how positive the outcome would be? Isn't it worth having a go and finding out?

'I feel overwhelmed'

Don't be hard on yourself. Making changes can seem daunting, especially if you have a lot to make at once – and I know there's a lot in this book to take in. Work on one Pillar at a time.

The Five Ps: Prior Planning Prevents Poor Performance

This has become our family motto. When I first met my husband, I was anything but organized. Dinner time would roll around and I would realize that the food I wanted to cook had either not been bought yet or was still sitting in the freezer. It wasn't just meal prep, I was disorganized generally. When I asked how he managed to make family days out and the like run so smoothly, he replied, 'It's the Five Ps: Prior Planning Prevents Poor Performance'. That totally resonated with me and I started to implement it personally and with clients.

Plan ahead – Each week on Wednesdays or Thursdays look ahead to the meals and recipes coming in the following week and ensure you have all the ingredients that you need.

Do your shopping online – Avoid wasting time and energy on long queues and getting frustrated walking around the supermarket by placing an order online and having it delivered. Use that extra time to prep your meals.

Sunday cook off – Set time aside to batch cook items like granola or bone broth. Make and freeze sauces and soups in portion-size containers. Chop your smoothie ingredients and pop into portion-sized bags for the fridge or freezer. Following my meal plan? I have listed which items you can prep in advance.

Invest in a slow cooker – One of my favourite kitchen helpers! Easy to use and a time saver – pop in all the ingredients and come back to a sumptuous and warming meal a few hours later. I make bone broth overnight in my slow cooker and eat some for breakfast the next day.

Get the family involved – Enrol some chopping, packing and sorting helpers to help share the load.

What Happens Next?

You may be wondering (or worrying) about what you'll do when you've finished the four-week meal plan. First of all, congratulate yourself! You've made a big commitment to a new lifestyle, a balanced new you. I'm willing to bet you'll feel so fabulous that reverting to your old eating habits won't even cross your mind.

You'll have a wide new recipe repertoire to choose from for future meals. And you'll have a good understanding and working knowledge of all the principles of the plan. I'm confident you'll be able to move forwards and create your own deliciously balanced meals and snacks.

Can I Still Eat Out?

Absolutely! Most restaurants have healthy options and any good establishment will answer questions or allow you to tweak dishes to suit your dietary requirements. You can always call ahead to ask about gluten- or dairy-free options, too. Relax and enjoy your night out and make the best choice with what you have available to you. Remember the 80/20 rule, too – it's not about perfection. Some useful rules:

— skip the bread basket and go for olives
— order a side salad
— ask for a jug or bottle of water, especially if you're going to have some wine
— plain grilled fish, chicken or meat are good options
— order extra vegetables instead of fries
— stir-fries and coconut- or tomato-based curries with gluten-free noodles or with rice are good choices
— avoid fried food and creamy sauce dishes
— for dessert, see if there is a fruit option

SOS Food for Snack Attacks

We have all been there: suddenly hungry with nothing to hand. Maybe you're stuck in traffic, had to work through lunch or your train is delayed. Maybe you're just peckish for a snack and want to ensure you've a healthy choice to hand. I always have an 'SOS' food pack with me in a little cooler bag. It might include any of the following:

— single serving almond butter packs
— an apple
— small bag of almonds or mixed nuts
— small pouch of olives
— veggie sticks
— hummus
— small can of no-drain fish
— biltong or jerky (I was born and raised in sunny south Africa!)
— water
— hard-boiled eggs
— oatcakes
— falafel
— piece of fruit
— small bottle of kefir
— small tub of three-bean salad
— miso soup or bone broth
— sliced chicken or turkey breast
— pieces of fresh coconut

Reintroducing Certain Foods

I get it, not everyone wants to be gluten and dairy free. But if you want to bring them back, I recommend having a gluten- and dairy-light diet. Don't have them every day and at every meal; instead only have them a couple of times a week and alternate the type of gluten and dairy sources you are having.

Gluten

Vary it with sourdough, rye, spelt, durum, pearl barley, semolina and other grains.

Dairy

Go for organic and swap in goats' and sheep dairy, too.

Mantras to Live by

Temptation in your way? Breathe deep and remember…
— I make the best decision I can with what is available to me
— The Six Pillars to hormonal freedom are my foundation
— I follow the Balance Plan 80/20 rule
— I live by the 'Five Ps' motto
— Fat isn't the enemy, sugar is
— My body loves balance and movement
— I have protein with every meal and snack
— When life is crazy I find a moment of calm, just for me

It's a good idea to reintroduce these common trigger foods one at a time: have it twice during one day, then wait 72 hours to see if you have a reaction. Reactions may mean anything from digestive complaints like bloating, burping, flatulence and bowel-function change to headaches, fatigue and skin reactions. If you suspect a reaction, I would recommend seeing a registered nutritional therapist or your health care practitioner.

Caffeine

Can't live without your beloved coffee or tea? I would recommend that you limit it to one cup a day or every couple of days, and no sugar.

Alcohol

The rule of thumb for drinking alcohol is to keep it to your 20 per cent and only have good-quality alcohol like a good-quality dry red wine (highest in antioxidants) or a clear spirit, such as vodka, with sparkling water and fresh lime. No cheap sugary booze and mixers that will send your Sassy Six into a spin. Limit it to one night a week with no more than two units consumed. Special occasion? OK, but rein it in again afterwards!

Sugar

By now you know that sugar is the enemy of hormonal balance. Keep sugar to your 20 per cent and favour natural forms like honey and maple syrup in moderation. Trust me, your tastebuds will change and you won't want the white stuff.

Meal Plan: Week One

Pre-week Sunday cook off: Chicken Stock (*see* page 166), Purple Coleslaw
(*see* page 195), Spinach & Cashew Pesto (*see* page 199), Hummus of choice
(*see* page 188), Simple Sauerkraut (*see* page 200), Vegetable Frittata (*see* page 130),
Blueberry Chia Jam (*see* page 119), Smoothie bags (*see* pages 108–110)

	BREAKFAST	LUNCH
MONDAY *Prepare salad for lunch and breakfast for the morning*	Berry Breakfast Porridge (*see* page 114) Wake-up Smoothie (*see* page 110)	Vegetable Frittata & Speedy Salad (*see* page 130) *Prepared the night before*
TUESDAY *Prepare lunch for tomorrow*	Coconut Chia Porridge & Blueberry Chia Jam (*see* page 119) Green Boost Smoothie (*see* page 109)	Chicken Salad (*see* page 157)
WEDNESDAY *Prepare breakfast and lunch for tomorrow*	Energy Eggs (*see* page 128) Smoothie of choice (*see* pages 108–110)	Flaked Salmon Sandwich with Purple Coleslaw (*see* pages 142 and 195)
THURSDAY *Prepare lunch for tomorrow*	Raw Oat, Fruit & Nut Porridge (see page 114) Green Machine Smoothie (*see* page 110)	Chicken & Vegetable Stir-fry with Rainbow Salad (*see* pages 162 and 192)
FRIDAY *Prepare lunch for tomorrow*	Quinoa & Berry Porridge (*see* page 116) Green Machine Smoothie (*see* page 110)	Butter Bean & Courgetti Salad (*see* page 179)
SATURDAY *Prepare lunch for tomorrow*	Mini Oat Pancakes (*see* page 127) Beetroot Smoothie (*see* page 110)	Pesto & Almond-crumbed Cod with Minty Peas and Chop Chop Salad (*see* pages 140 and 192)
SUNDAY *Start prepping your lamb wraps for tomorrow*	The Best Brunch (*see* page 126) Smoothie of choice (*see* pages 108–110)	Cauliflower Pizza with Rainbow Salad (*see* pages 160 and 192)

DINNER	SNACKS (only if needed)	LIFESTYLE TIPS
Lemon & Rosemary Chicken with Purple Coleslaw (*see* pages 156 and 195)	Hummus and veggie sticks (*see* page 188)	Plan ahead and follow the Five Ps (*see* page 95) – look ahead to the next day and see what you need to prepare in advance
Lemon & Dill Salmon with Cauliflower Mash (*see* page 150)		Stop and breathe if things start to feel overwhelming
Chicken & Vegetable Stir-fry with Rainbow Salad (*see* pages 162 and 192)	Chop Chop Salad (*see* page 192) and a mug of bone broth	Snack only when you are actually hungry, and choose snacks that will help maintain your energy levels and stave off those hunger pangs
Butter Bean & Courgetti Salad (*see* page 179)	Red Pepper Hummus and veggie sticks (*see* page 188)	Have a look at the week ahead and buy all the ingredients needed
Pesto & Almond-crumbed Cod with Minty Peas and Chop Chop Salad (*see* pages 140 and 192)	Boiled egg and olives	Eat some Sauerkraut (*see* page 200) as a condiment to your evening meal
Cauliflower Pizza with Rainbow Salad (*see* pages 160 and 192)	Handful of nuts and seeds, and a Spiced Matcha Latte (*see* page 112)	Schedule in some 'me time' and stick to it
Slow-cooked Lamb & Roots with Steamed Greens and Creamy Salad (*see* pages 198, 196 and 176)	Pesto (*see* page 199) and veggie sticks	Download a period tracker to keep tabs on your cycle (*see* page 34)

Meal Plan: Week Two

Pre-week Sunday cook off: Spiced Sweet Potato & Carrot Granola (*see* page 120),
Pistachio Pesto (*see* page 199), Crispy Roasted Chickpeas (*see* page 186),
Blueberry Chia Jam (*see* page 119), Smoothie bags (*see* pages 108–110)

	BREAKFAST	LUNCH
MONDAY *Prepare lunch for tomorrow*	Spiced Sweet Potato & Carrot Granola (*see* page 120) Tropical Turmeric Smoothie (*see* page 108)	Lamb & Creamy Salad Wraps (*see* page 176)
TUESDAY *Make Coconut Chia Porridge (see page 119)*	Eggs, Avocado & Tomato on Wilted Spinach (*see* page 122) Smoothie of choice (*see* pages 108–110)	Coconut-crumbed Chicken with Cauliflower Mash and Mixed Herb Salad (*see* pages 171, 150 and 191)
WEDNESDAY *Prepare lunch for tomorrow*	Coconut Chia Porridge & Blueberry Chia Jam (*see* page 119) Green Boost Smoothie (*see* page 109)	Lentil & Quinoa Sweet Potato Burgers (*see* page 138)
THURSDAY *Prepare lunch for tomorrow*	Energy Eggs (*see* page 128) Smoothie of choice (*see* pages 108–110)	Thai-style Prawn & Mussel Stir-fry (*see* page 153)
FRIDAY *Prepare lunch for tomorrow*	Spiced Sweet Potato & Carrot Granola (*see* page 120) Tropical Turmeric Smoothie (*see* page 108)	Cauliflower, Beetroot & Chickpea Wraps with Mixed Herb Salad (*see* pages 136 and 191)
SATURDAY *Prepare lunch for tomorrow*	Mini Oat Pancakes (*see* page 127) Blueberry & Macadamia Smoothie (*see* page 108)	Grilled Salmon with Broad Bean & Pesto Mash (*see* page 144)
SUNDAY *Prepare lunch for tomorrow*	The Best Brunch (*see* page 126) Spiced Matcha Latte (*see* page 112)	Chunky Chicken Soup (*see* page 166)

DINNER	SNACKS (only if needed)	LIFESTYLE TIPS
Coconut-crumbed Chicken with Cauliflower Mash and Mixed Herb Salad (*see* pages 171, 150 and 191)	Crispy Roasted Chickpeas (*see* page 186)	Do your 4/7 breathing (*see* page 68) for a calm, focussed start to your week
Lentil & Quinoa Sweet Potato Burgers (*see* page 138)		Choose an affirmation (*see* page 80) to start your day with
Thai-style Prawn & Mussel Stir-fry (*see* page 153)	Fruit Salad & Coconut Yogurt (*see* page 208)	Remember to stay hydrated
Cauliflower, Beetroot & Chickpea Wraps with Mixed Herb Salad (*see* pages 136 and 191)		Have a look at the week ahead and buy all the ingredients needed
Grilled Salmon with Broad Bean & Pesto Mash (*see* page 144)	Pesto (*see* page 199) and veggie sticks	Get to bed a little earlier and have a good night's rest
Slow-cooked Roast Chicken & Veg with Chop Chop Salad (*see* pages 178 and 192)	Smoothie of choice (*see* pages 108–110)	Organise a girly catch-up and get some laughs in
Turkey Meatballs & Butternut 'Spaghetti' with salad or greens of choice (*see* pages 158, 191–192 and 196–198)	Handful of nuts and seeds Smoothie of choice (*see* pages 108–110)	Get some movement in today by trying out a new activity

Meal Plan: Week Three

Pre-week Sunday cook off: Crispy Roasted Chickpeas (*see* page 186), Hummus of choice (*see* page 188), Pesto of choice (*see* page 199), Chicken or vegetable stock as needed (*see* page 166), Almond & Cashew Protein Balls (*see* page 202), Simple Sauerkraut (*see* page 200), Blueberry Chia Jam (*see* page 119), Smoothie bags (*see* pages 108–110)

	BREAKFAST	LUNCH
MONDAY *Take out a portion of Chicken Soup*	Eggs, Avocado & Tomato on Wilted Spinach (*see* page 122) Wake-up Smoothie (*see* page 110)	Turkey Meatballs & Butternut 'Spaghetti' with salad or greens of choice (*see* pages 158, 191–192 and 196–198)
TUESDAY *Prepare lunch for tomorrow*	Cinnamon Millet Porridge (*see* page 116) Green Nutrition Smoothie (*see* page 110)	Sea Bass Parcels with Dill & Capers with Minty Peas and Steamed Greens (*see* pages 148, 140 and 198)
WEDNESDAY *Prepare lunch for tomorrow*	Energy Eggs (*see* page 128) Smoothie of choice (*see* pages 108–110)	Vegetarian Pad Thai (*see* page 143)
THURSDAY *Portion lunch*	Spiced Sweet Potato & Carrot Granola (*see* page 120) Tropical Turmeric Smoothie (*see* page 108)	Chicken Fajita Wraps (*see* page 165)
FRIDAY *Prepare lunch for tomorrow*	Quinoa & Berry Porridge (*see* page 116) Green Machine Smoothie (*see* page 110)	Turkey Burgers & Tandoori-roasted Cauliflower with Mixed Herb Salad (*see* pages 182 and 191)
SATURDAY *Prepare lunch for tomorrow*	Eggs, Avocado & Tomato on Wilted Spinach (*see* page 122) Green Nutrition Smoothie (*see* page 110)	Stuffed Sweet Potato with Steamed Greens (*see* pages 135 and 198)
SUNDAY *Prepare breakfast and lunch for tomorrow*	Buckwheat & Smoked Salmon Pancakes (*see* page 124) Blueberry & Macadamia Smoothie (*see* page 108)	Lemon & Dill Salmon with Cauliflower Mash and Chop Chop Salad (*see* pages 150 and 192)

DINNER	SNACKS (only if needed)	LIFESTYLE TIPS
Sea Bass Parcels with Dill & Capers with Minty Peas and Steamed Greens (*see* pages 148, 140 and 198)	Smoothie of choice (*see* pages 108–110)	Start your week off with the attitude of gratitude – what are you thankful for?
Vegetarian Pad Thai (*see* page 143)	Chunky Chicken Soup (*see* page 166)	Lunch in the park? Brisk walk to work? Get outside and soak up some of that natural daylight
Chicken Fajita Wraps (*see* page 165) Simple Sauerkraut (*see* page 200)	Pear with almond butter	Check your poo against the chart on page 48 to see if you are popping perfect poos yet
Turkey Burgers & Tandoori-roasted Cauliflower with Mixed Herb Salad (*see* pages 182 and 191)	Crispy Roasted Chickpeas (*see* page 186)	Have a look at the week ahead and buy all the ingredients needed
Stuffed Sweet Potato with Steamed Greens (*see* pages 135 and 198)	Handful of nuts and seeds	Breakfast is king: schedule in enough time in the morning to eat well
Lemon & Dill Salmon with Cauliflower Mash and Chop Chop Salad (*see* pages 150 and 192)	Mug of chicken or vegetable broth (experiment with other bones, too)	Try a yoga class
Satay-style Chicken with Cauliflower Rice and Mixed Herb Salad (*see* pages 155 and 191)	Baked Apples with Vanilla Cashew Cream (*see* page 204)	Make time for a long Epsom-salt bath soak to unwind (*see* page 74)

Meal Plan: Week Four

Pre-week Sunday cook off: Crispy Roasted Chickpeas (*see* page 186), Hummus of choice (*see* page 188), Pesto of choice (*see* page 199), Chicken or vegetable stock as needed (*see* page 166), Blueberry Chia Jam (*see* page 119), Smoothie bags (*see* pages 108–110)

	BREAKFAST	LUNCH
MONDAY *Prepare lunch for tomorrow*	Coconut Chia Porridge & Blueberry Chia Jam (*see* page 119) Green Boost Smoothie (*see* page 109)	Satay-style Chicken with Cauliflower Rice and Mixed Herb Salad (*see* pages 155 and 191)
TUESDAY *Pack lunch for tomorrow*	Eggs, Avocado & Tomato on Wilted Spinach (*see* page 122) Green Nutrition Smoothie (*see* page 110)	Steak Strip Stir-fry (*see* page 180)
WEDNESDAY *Pack lunch for tomorrow*	Spiced Sweet Potato & Carrot Granola (*see* page 120) Tropical Turmeric Smoothie (*see* page 108)	Zesty Turkey Pasta Salad (*see* page 168)
THURSDAY *Pack lunch for tomorrow*	Energy Eggs (*see* page 128) Smoothie of choice (*see* pages 108–110)	Pan-roast Halibut with Artichokes & Broccoli (*see* page 146)
FRIDAY *Prep breakfast for tomorrow*	Quinoa & Berry Porridge (*see* page 116) Green Machine Smoothie (*see* page 110)	Lentil & Quinoa Sweet Potato Burgers with Thai Mango Salad (*see* pages 138 and 132)
SATURDAY *Prepare lunch for tomorrow*	Raw Oat, Fruit & Nut Porridge (*see* page 114) Green Machine Smoothie (*see* page 110)	Thai-style Prawn & Mussel Stir-fry (*see* page 153)
SUNDAY *Prepare lunch for tomorrow*	The Best Brunch (*see* page 126) Smoothie of choice (*see* pages 108–110)	Chicken Salad (*see* page 157)

DINNER	SNACKS (only if needed)	LIFESTYLE TIPS
Steak Strip Stir-fry (*see* page 180)	Pesto (*see* page 199) and veggie sticks	Chew your food well – 20 to 30 chews per mouthful – your stomach doesn't have teeth
Zesty Turkey Pasta Salad (*see* page 168)	Handful of nuts and seeds	Start the day with some dry brushing (*see* pages 74–75)
Pan-roast Halibut with Artichokes & Broccoli (*see* page 146)	Apple and almond nut butter with a sprinkle of cinnamon	Stave off cravings with a mug of cinnamon tea
Lentil & Quinoa Sweet Potato Burgers with Thai Mango Salad (*see* pages 138 and 132)		Have a look at the week ahead and buy all the ingredients needed
Thai-style Prawn & Mussel Stir-fry (*see* page 153)	Mini Oat Pancakes (*see* page 127), oatcakes or brown rice cakes with guacamole	Get some movement in
Slow-cooked Roast Chicken & Veg with Chop Chop Salad (*see* pages 178 and 192)	Smoothie of choice (*see* pages 108–110)	Look back at your food diary – what changes can you see between you then and the you now?
Rich Lamb Curry with Steamed Greens (*see* pages 172 and 198)	Spiced Matcha Latte (*see* page 112)	Write down your body measurements – how do they compare with those that you took at the start of the plan?

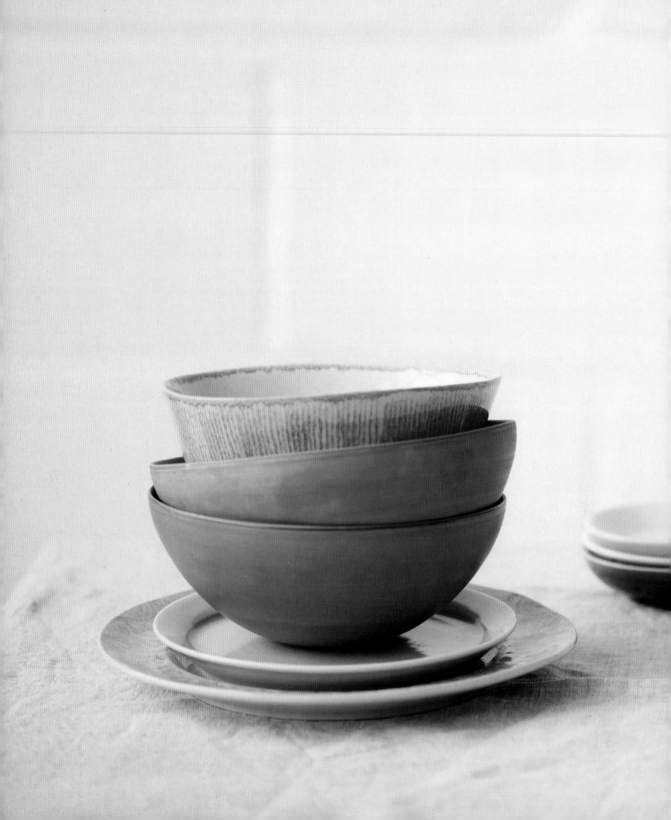

recipes

Blueberry & Macadamia Smoothie

This pretty little wonder is full of healthy fats and hormone-healing goodness.

<u>1 serving</u>

80g (2³/₄oz) blueberries, fresh or frozen

2 handfuls of spinach

30g (1oz) macadamia nuts, preferably pre-soaked

200ml (7fl oz) unsweetened almond milk

¹/₂ teaspoon ground cinnamon

¹/₂ teaspoon turmeric

1 teaspoon maca powder

a pinch of ground black pepper

Put all the ingredients into a blender with 100ml (3¹/₂fl oz) of water and blend well, adding more water or almond milk if you need to. Serve immediately.

Tropical Turmeric Smoothie

Earthy turmeric, one of nature's great healers, is perfect for adding a supercharged boost.

<u>1 serving</u>

2 small handfuls of kale or spinach

200ml (7fl oz) coconut milk

100g (3¹/₂oz) pineapple, including the core

¹/₄ unwaxed lemon (skin optional)

1cm (¹/₂ inch) piece of fresh ginger, skin on

1 teaspoon ground turmeric, or to taste

¹/₂ teaspoon ground cinnamon

¹/₄ teaspoon ground black pepper

¹/₂ teaspoon coconut oil

Put all the ingredients into a blender and blend well, adding water or more coconut milk if you need to. Serve immediately.

Green Boost Smoothie

A good combo of antioxidants, essential fats and fibre, while ginger aids digestion and reduces inflammation.

1 serving

120g (4^1/$_4$oz) baby spinach leaves
^{1}/$_2$ cucumber, chopped
a small handful of fresh flat-leaf parsley
^{1}/$_2$ pineapple, peeled and cubed, including the core
^{1}/$_4$ avocado
^{1}/$_2$ unwaxed lemon (skin optional)
1cm (^{1}/$_2$ inch) piece of fresh ginger, skin on
2 teaspoons ground flax seeds

Put all the ingredients into a blender with 200–250ml (7–9fl oz) of water and blend well, adding more water if you need to. Serve immediately.

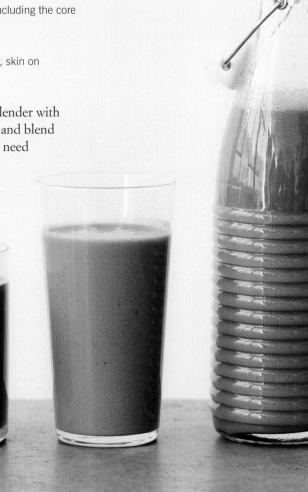

Green Machine

With avocado and flax seeds, this smoothie is full of hormone-balancing good fats.

1 serving

3 handfuls of kale or spinach
2 sticks of celery
1/4 avocado
a small handful of fresh flat-leaf parsley
1 teaspoon ground flax seeds
1/4 unwaxed lemon or lime (skin optional)
1 teaspoon of your favourite superfood powder (optional)

Put all the ingredients into a blender with 250ml (9fl oz) of water and blend well, adding more water if you need to. Serve immediately.

Beetroot Smoothie

Beautiful beets are one of nature's best detoxifiers. This cleanses from the inside, out.

1 serving

1–2 small beetroots
1 carrot
1/2 apple
a handful of baby spinach
1/4 teaspoon coconut oil
1cm (1/2 inch) piece of fresh ginger
a squeeze of lemon juice
2 tablespoons ground flax seeds

Put all the ingredients into a blender with 250ml (9fl oz) of water and blend well, adding more water if you need to. Serve immediately.

Green Nutrition

If you love a healthy smoothie kick, then this is perfect for you.

1 serving

2 handfuls of kale
2 sticks of celery
1/4 cucumber
1 apple
1/2 unwaxed lemon (skin optional)
2cm (3/4 inch) piece of fresh ginger, skin on
1/4 avocado
2 teaspoons ground flax seeds

Put all the ingredients into a blender with 250ml (9fl oz) of water and blend well, adding more water if you need to. Serve immediately.

Wake-up Smoothie

In need of a pick-me-up? Step away from the coffee and whizz up one of these instead.

1 serving

1/2–1 teaspoon matcha powder
1/2 avocado
a handful of baby spinach
1 teaspoon coconut oil
2 tablespoons ground flax seeds
1/4 teaspoon ground cinnamon
1 apple
1/4 unwaxed lemon (skin optional)
1 teaspoon of your favourite superfood powder (optional)

Put all the ingredients into a blender with 250ml (9fl oz) of water and blend well, adding more water if you need to. Serve immediately.

Berry & Mint Fizz

This fruity fizz is like nature's very own cocktail and it's full of berry beautiful antioxidants.

Makes 1 litre (1³/₄ pints)

100g (3¹/₂oz) mixed berries
1 litre (1³/₄ pints) sparkling water
a small handful of fresh mint leaves
ice

Crush the berries lightly in a bowl to extract some of their juices, then spoon them into a jug of sparkling water.

Add mint leaves to taste.

Add ice and leave to infuse in the fridge for about 30 minutes.

Mint & Cucumber Cooler

I love adding cucumber to water because it's so hydrating and refreshing.

Makes 1 litre (1³/₄ pints)

¹/₂ organic cucumber, washed
1 unwaxed organic lemon, washed
1 litre (1³/₄ pints) sparkling water
a small handful of fresh mint leaves
ice

Use a vegetable peeler to slice the cucumber into ribbons.

Cut the lemon in half. Squeeze the juice of one half into a jug of sparkling water, then cut the other half into slices and add them to the jug.

Add mint leaves to taste.

Add ice and leave to infuse in the fridge for about 30 minutes.

Spiced Matcha Latte

This sweet and creamy drink will give you all the rocket fuel you need in the morning – without needing to reach for coffee. Matcha powder is full of antioxidants, can help promote a sense of calm and detoxify your hormones.

<u>1 serving</u>

1 teaspoon matcha powder

200ml (7fl oz) filtered water, half of it at room temperature and half of it hot

200ml (7fl oz) coconut milk

1/4 teaspoon vanilla powder

1/4 teaspoon ground cinnamon

1/4 teaspoon ground nutmeg

1/2 teaspoon turmeric

a pinch of ground black pepper

1 teaspoon raw honey (optional)

Blitz all the ingredients, except the hot water, in a blender for 30–40 seconds, or until well combined.

Pour in the hot water and blend again.

Serve as a warm drink, or pour over ice, sprinkling with more cinnamon if you like.

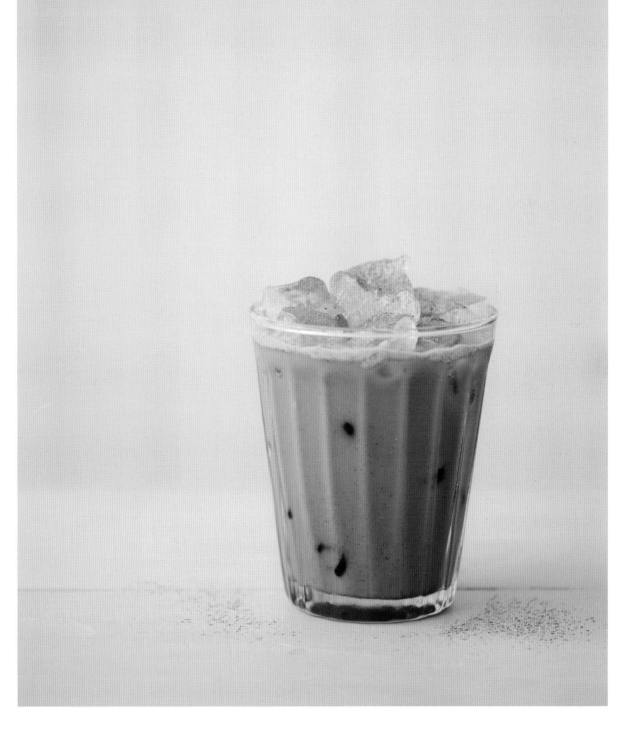

Raw Oat, Fruit & Nut Porridge (pictured)

Say goodbye to those sugar-rich breakfast cereals – you really don't need them. This raw porridge is full of fibre, protein and essential fats to set your hormone patterns for the day. Start preparing it the night before – every minute counts in the morning.

1 serving

4 tablespoons gluten-free jumbo oat flakes

1/2 teaspoon ground cinnamon

1 tablespoon pumpkin seeds

1 tablespoon sunflower seeds

200ml (7fl oz) unsweetened or homemade almond milk

1 tablespoon pecan nuts, roughly chopped

1 tablespoon hazelnuts, roughly chopped

2 tablespoons ground flax seeds

80g (2³/4oz) mixed berries

Mix the oats, cinnamon and pumpkin and sunflower seeds in a bowl. Add the milk, stir well, then cover and refrigerate overnight.

By morning, the mixture should have soaked up most of the milk. Add the nuts, ground flax seeds and berries to the oat mixture and combine well.

Serve with more milk and extra cinnamon, if desired.

Berry Breakfast Porridge

This is a wholesome, healthy twist on a breakfast classic, and comes with plenty of added goodness. Better still, the crunchy nuts add fats and protein to keep you full all morning.

1 serving

45g (1¹/2oz) gluten-free jumbo oats

230ml (8fl oz) coconut milk or almond milk, plus extra to serve

100g (3¹/2oz) mixed berries, fresh or frozen

45g (1¹/2oz) raw, finely chopped nuts and seeds

a sprinkling of ground cinnamon

Put the oats and milk into a saucepan with 230ml (8fl oz) of water and bring to the boil, stirring continuously. Allow to simmer on a low to medium heat for 15–20 minutes, stirring occasionally.

Meanwhile, put the berries into a blender and blitz to a purée – you may need to add a little water. Set aside.

Transfer the cooked oats to a bowl and spoon over the fruit purée. Sprinkle over the nuts and seeds and serve, adding a splash of extra milk and a sprinkling of cinnamon.

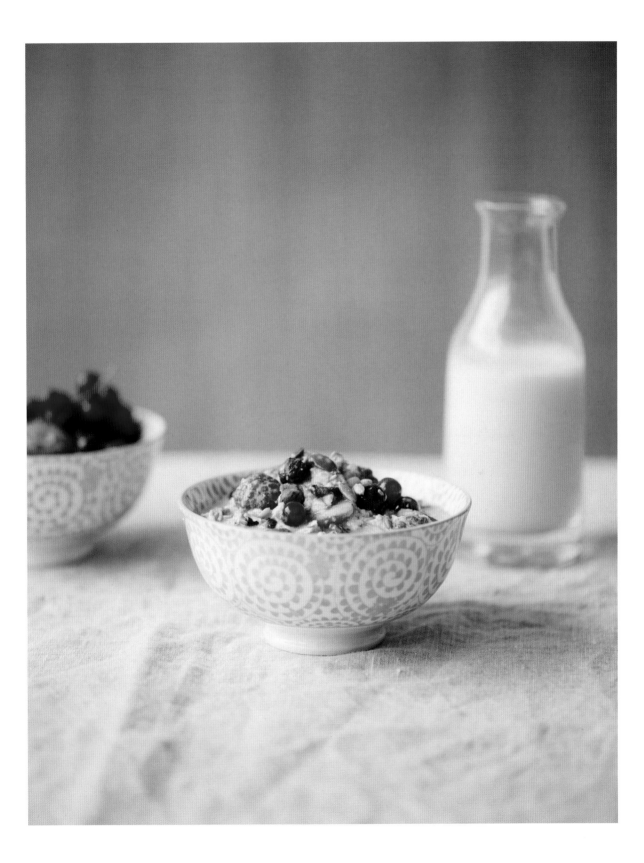

Quinoa & Berry Porridge (pictured)

This makes a great alternative to sugar-laden breakfast cereals, and is high in protein too. The perfect way to kickstart your day.

1 serving

80g (2³/₄oz) cooked quinoa

120ml (3³/₄fl oz) coconut milk or almond milk, plus extra to drizzle

¹/₂ teaspoon ground cinnamon

1 tablespoon shredded coconut (unsweetened)

¹/₂ teaspoon vanilla powder

20g (³/₄oz) flaked almonds

a pinch of sea salt

1–2 tablespoons coconut yogurt

2 tablespoons maca powder

1 teaspoon pumpkin seeds

30g (1oz) thawed frozen berries, or fresh berries

Combine the quinoa, milk, cinnamon, coconut, vanilla, almonds and salt in a small saucepan over a medium heat. Cook, stirring for 5–6 minutes, until the milk has been absorbed and the porridge reaches a creamy consistency.

Spoon into a serving bowl, drizzling with extra milk if desired.

Top with the yogurt, maca powder, pumpkin seeds and berries and serve.

Cinnamon Millet Porridge

This fibre-rich millet porridge is ideal morning rocket fuel, while the addition of naturally sweet cinnamon can help your body to balance out blood-sugar levels.

1 serving

100ml (3¹/₂fl oz) coconut milk

50g (1³/₄oz) millet flakes

1 teaspoon ground cinnamon

1 teaspoon coconut oil

zest of ¹/₂ orange

1 teaspoon desiccated coconut

3 tablespoons mixed seeds

1 teaspoon chia seeds

Put the coconut milk into a saucepan with 100ml (3¹/₂fl oz) of water and bring to the boil.

Add the millet flakes and simmer until cooked and creamy for approximately 15 minutes. If it is too thick, add some water or milk.

Remove from the heat and stir in the cinnamon, chia seeds and coconut oil. Sprinkle the coconut, zest and seeds on top and serve.

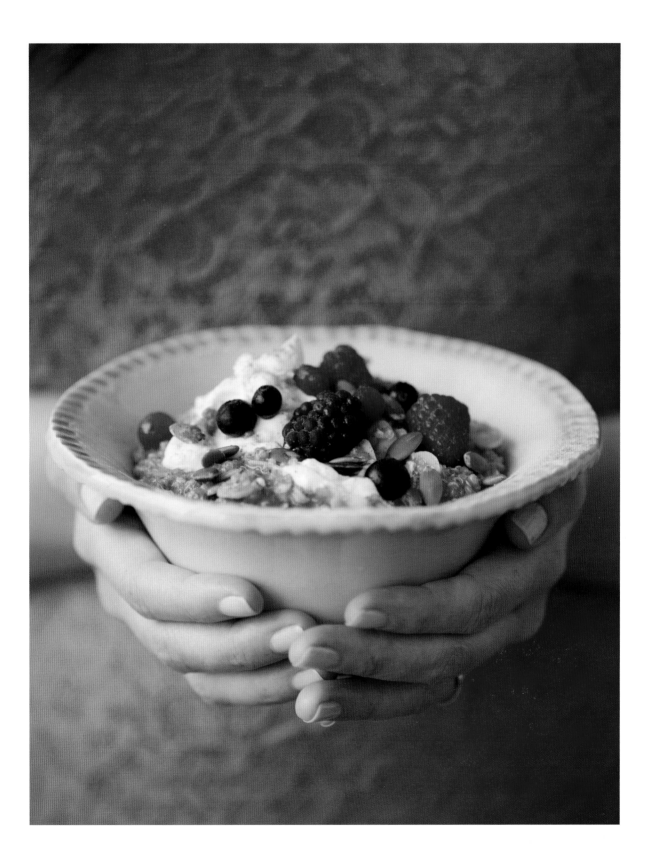

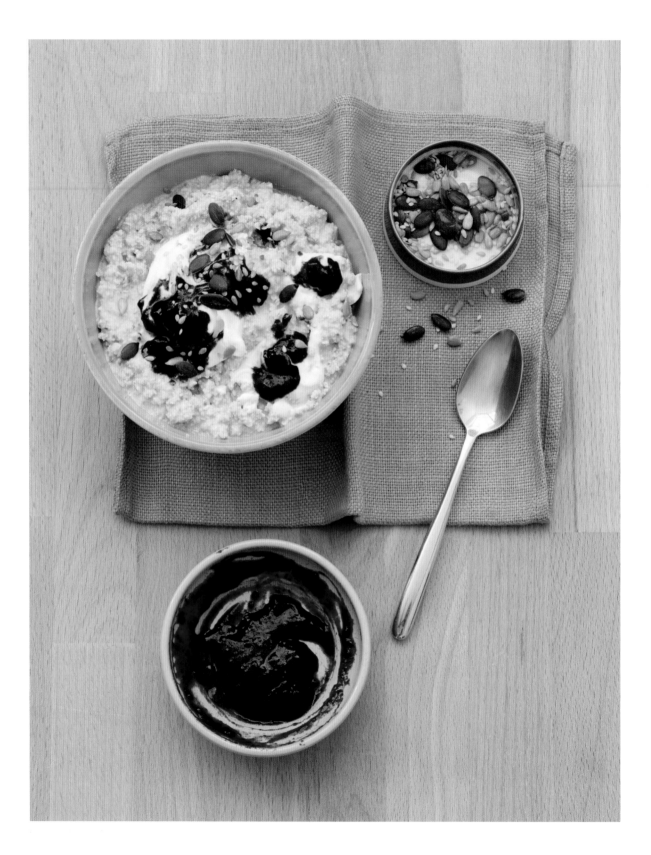

Coconut Chia Porridge & Blueberry Chia Jam

Chia seeds are an ancient grain that contain huge amounts of fibre and omega-3, and they can ease blood-sugar spikes too. Blueberries are rich in vitamin C, potassium and fibre. This chia jam also tastes delicious spread on toast or rice cakes.

2 servings

For the blueberry chia jam
400g (14oz) blueberries, fresh or frozen
1–2 dates, stoned
1/2 teaspoon vanilla paste
juice of 1/2 lemon
2 tablespoons chia seeds

For the porridge
80g (2 3/4oz) desiccated coconut
12 almonds
450ml (16fl oz) dairy-free milk of choice
juice of 1/2 lemon
2 tablespoons ground almonds
1 1/2 teaspoons vanilla paste
a pinch of salt
2 teaspoons maca powder
2 tablespoons chia seeds

To serve
2 tablespoons blueberry chia jam
  (*see* above)
2 tablespoons coconut yogurt
2 tablespoons mixed seeds

First, make the blueberry jam. Put the blueberries into a saucepan (add 1 tablespoon of water if using fresh). Gently heat, stirring often, until the skins break down and they form a purée. Remove from the heat. Put into a blender with the dates and vanilla paste and blitz to your desired consistency.

Stir in the lemon juice and chia seeds, then allow to cool – the mixture will thicken over time and will be ready for spreading after a couple of hours. Pour into an airtight glass jar and store in the fridge for up to 1 week. You can also freeze the jam in ice-cube trays – perfect for popping straight into smoothies.

Stir together all the ingredients for the porridge, apart from the chia seeds, in a large bowl. Transfer to a blender and blitz until smooth and creamy, or until you reach your desired consistency.

Stir the chia seeds through the porridge, then cover and refrigerate overnight.

Serve hot or cold the next day, with spoonfuls of blueberry chia jam and coconut yogurt, and a sprinkling of mixed seeds.

Spiced Sweet Potato & Carrot Granola

This deliciously spiced granola gets its sweetness from fibrous sweet potatoes and carrots, which will keep your blood sugars from spiking. Meanwhile, healing cinnamon can also balance out your insulin. A breakfast of champions.

8–10 servings

150g (5½oz) sweet potatoes, chopped
100g (3½oz) carrots, chopped
1 tablespoon coconut oil
¼ teaspoon ground cloves
¼ teaspoon ground ginger
¼ teaspoon ground nutmeg
1 teaspoon ground cinnamon
2 teaspoons vanilla extract
a pinch of sea salt
80g (2¾oz) unsweetened coconut flakes
100g (3½oz) ground almonds
100g (3½oz) sliced almonds
100g (3½oz) pecans, chopped
80g (2¾oz) pumpkin seeds
80g (2¾oz) sunflower seeds
3 heaped tablespoons ground flax seeds

To serve

5 heaped tablespoons coconut yogurt, almond milk or coconut milk
½ teaspoon ground cinnamon
a small handful of blueberries

Preheat the oven to 180°C/350°F/gas mark 4. Line a large baking tray with baking paper, or grease the surface with a touch of coconut oil.

Steam the sweet potatoes and carrots until soft, for 15–20 minutes.

Once cooked, put the sweet potatoes and carrots into a high-powered blender, along with the coconut oil, cloves, ginger, nutmeg, cinnamon, vanilla extract and salt, and blend. You may need to add up to 220ml (8fl oz) of water if it's hard to blend, but be careful not to make the purée too watery. Allow the mixture to cool while you prepare the dry ingredients.

In a large bowl, combine the coconut flakes, ground and sliced almonds, pecans and seeds.

Add the wet ingredients from the blender to the dry ingredients and stir until well combined. The dry ingredients should be thoroughly coated.

Spread the granola in a thin layer on the prepared tray and bake for 20 minutes. Remove the tray from the oven and turn the granola to prevent it burning – oven temperatures can vary, so keep a close eye the first few times you make it.

Return to the oven, this time leaving the oven door open a few centimetres (an inch or two) – this will allow moisture from the oven to escape and will help crisp up the granola. Bake for a further 25–30 minutes, or until the granola is golden and crunchy.

Remove from the oven and allow to cool, then put into an airtight container and store for up to 2 weeks.

To serve, spoon 60g (2¼oz) of granola into a bowl. Top with the yogurt or milk, sprinkle with the cinnamon and blueberries, then eat and enjoy.

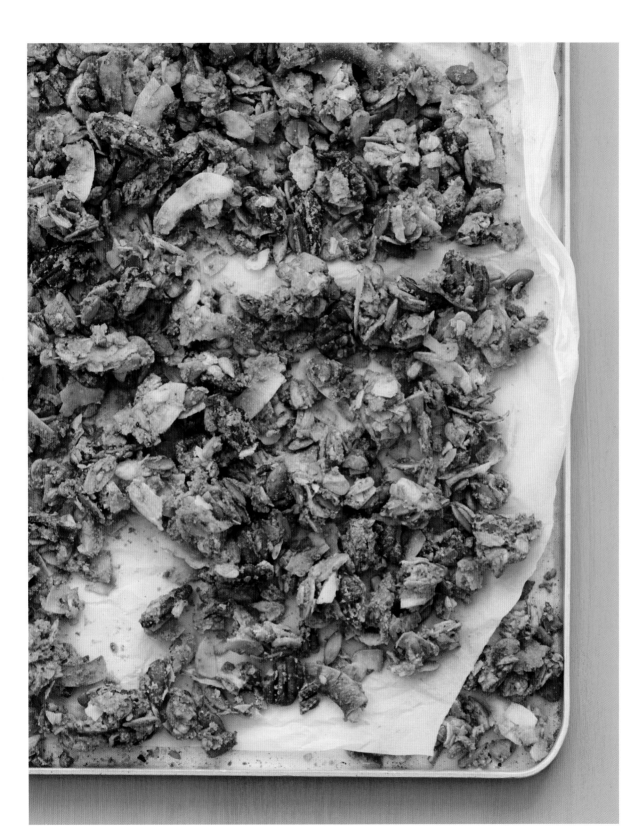

Eggs, Avocado & Tomato on Wilted Spinach

A quick and easy classic in our house, and one that should take no longer than 10 minutes from prep to table. Additional benefits? Spinach is jam-packed with vitamins and minerals, including iron, folic acid and vitamin C.

<u>1 serving</u>

2 organic free-range eggs
2 handfuls of fresh baby spinach
extra virgin olive oil
1 large vine tomato
1/2 ripe avocado, peeled and chopped
sea salt and black pepper

In a small saucepan, bring some cold water (enough to cover your eggs) to a rapid boil. Put in your eggs and let them boil to the texture you like. I aim for 5 minutes for a runny egg, 6 minutes for a soft-boiled egg, and 8 minutes for a hard-boiled egg.

Remove the eggs from the water with a slotted spoon and place on kitchen paper to dry.

Meanwhile, place the spinach in a separate saucepan on a medium heat. Add a dash of water, a drizzle of olive oil and some salt to taste, then cover with a lid and allow the spinach to wilt for 1–2 minutes. Remove from the pan and place on a plate.

Cut the tomato in half and place in the same saucepan, cut-side down. Add a drizzle of oil and sprinkle with sea salt. Keep on the heat for 1–2 minutes, until warm.

Deshell the eggs, place them on the bed of spinach and cut them in half. Add the tomato and avocado, sprinkle with salt and black pepper, and enjoy!

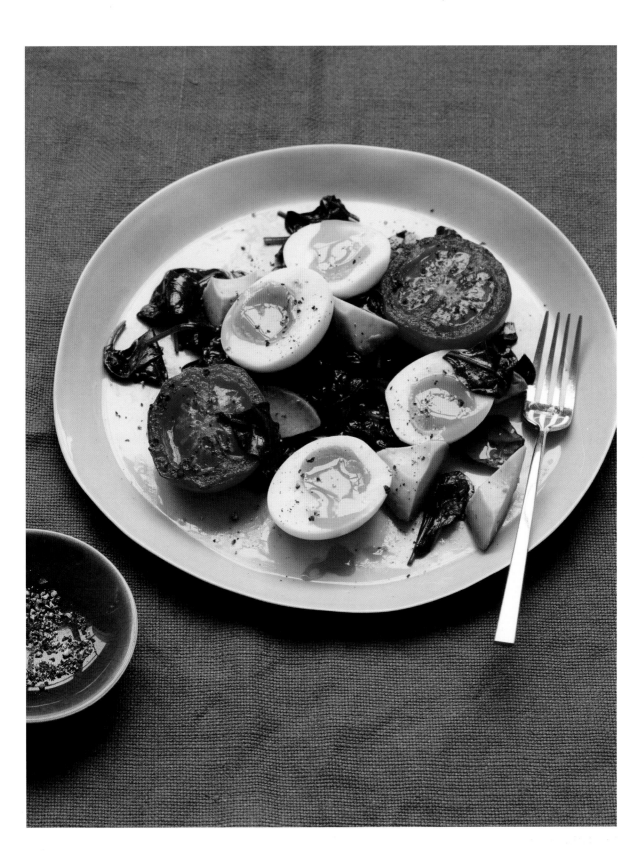

Buckwheat & Smoked Salmon Pancakes

Buckwheat, despite its name, is a naturally wheat-free grain and gives these pancakes a delicious nutty taste. Add some healthy fats and protein in the form of smoked salmon, and you're on to a breakfast winner.

2 servings
(makes 8 pancakes)

For the pancakes

355ml (12fl oz) water

220g (8oz) buckwheat flour

1 teaspoon aluminium and gluten-free baking powder

1/4 teaspoon cracked black pepper

1/2 teaspoon turmeric

1/2 teaspoon salt

3 tablespoons coconut oil

Toppings

1/2 pack of smoked salmon slices

1 large vine tomato, sliced

1 ripe avocado, peeled and chopped

a handful of fresh dill, chopped

1/2 lemon

Blend together all the pancake ingredients, except the coconut oil, to make a smooth batter.

Heat a little coconut oil in a non-stick frying pan. Add tablespoons of batter to the pan to form pancakes about 10cm (4 inches) across, you should be able to make 1–3 pancakes at a time, depending on the size of your pan. Cook for a couple of minutes, until you see bubbles appear on the top or you can easily peel the edges of the pancake away from the pan, then flip and cook on the other side until golden brown and cooked through.

Keep the pancakes warm while you finish cooking the remaining batter.

Serve stacked with smoked salmon, tomato slices and avocado, and sprinkle with dill and a squeeze of lemon.

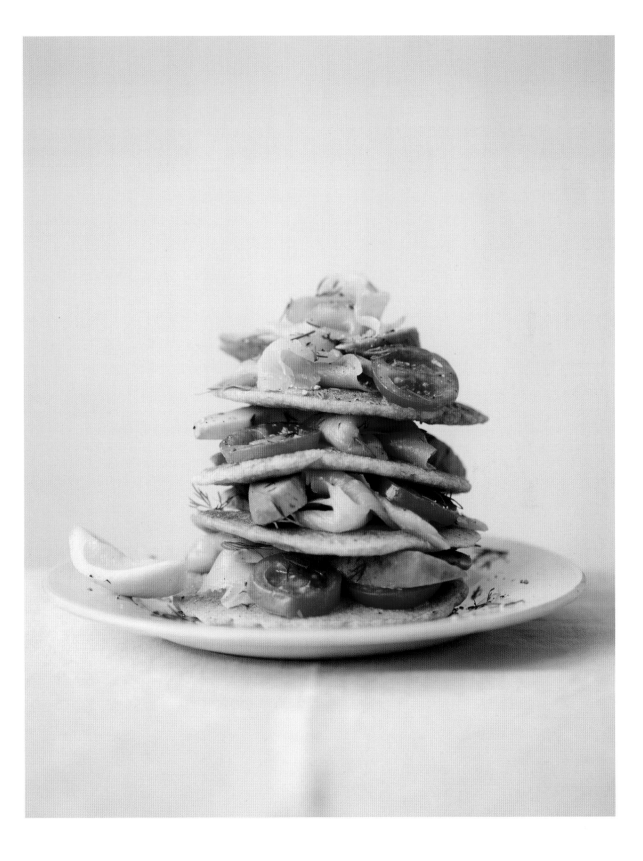

The Best Brunch

Poached eggs are one of those classic brunch dishes that always goes down a treat. With their gooey, delicious yolks, they work brilliantly with all sorts of foods. Here's my easy guide to the perfect plate.

1 serving

1 tablespoon extra virgin olive oil

2 vine-ripened tomatoes, cut into slices

2 handfuls of spinach

1 garlic clove, crushed

a splash of white vinegar

1 free-range organic egg, cracked into a small bowl or ramekin

½ ripe avocado, peeled and sliced

1 large slice of smoked salmon, cut into strips

2 teaspoons chopped fresh chives

salt and black pepper

Fill a small pan with enough water to cover an egg and bring it to the boil.

Meanwhile, heat a touch of olive oil in a frying pan. Add the tomatoes with a sprinkling of salt and pepper and cook for 5–6 minutes, stirring often, until they soften and their skins start to break down. Spoon the tomatoes on to a plate and place in a low oven to keep warm.

Using the same heated frying pan, add the spinach and garlic and sauté until the spinach has wilted. Set aside.

Return to your water, which should have boiled by now. Add the vinegar, give it a gentle swirl to create a whirlpool, then turn off the heat. Gently slide the egg from the bowl into the boiling water, then cover with a lid and leave until the egg white is completely opaque and the yolk is cooked to your liking (2–3 minutes or more if you're looking for a firmer yolk).

Remove the egg from the water using a slotted spoon, allowing the excess water to drain off, then place on kitchen paper to dry.

To serve, spoon the spinach on to a plate and top with the tomatoes and avocado. Carefully place the poached egg on top, then scatter over the smoked salmon, along with the chives and more salt and pepper, if desired. Eat immediately.

Mini Oat Pancakes

These oat and apple pancakes are delicious hot as a breakfast, but also taste great when served cold with a dollop of almond butter: the perfect snack to see you through a long afternoon.

2 servings

(makes 6–8 small pancakes)

For the batter

50g (1¾oz) gluten-free rolled oats

1 small red apple or pear, chopped

½ ripe banana

1 teaspoon aluminium and gluten-free baking powder

1 tablespoon ground flax seeds

1 teaspoon ground cinnamon

2 organic free-range eggs

a dash of coconut milk

1 tablespoon coconut oil or extra virgin olive oil

Toppings (optional)

coconut yogurt

almond butter, with grated apple or thinly sliced pear

blueberries

strawberries, halved

Place all the batter ingredients apart from ½ tablespoon of oil, into a blender and blend for a few minutes, or until the mixture forms a smooth batter. Let stand in the blender for 10–15 minutes, to thicken slightly.

Meanwhile, prepare the toppings.

When the batter is ready, heat the remaining ½ tablespoon of oil in a non-stick frying pan. Spoon in 1 tablespoon of batter for each small, circular pancake – you should be able to make 2–3 pancakes at a time, depending on the size of your pan. Lightly fry for 2–3 minutes, or until you can easily peel the edges of the pancake away from the pan, then flip and cook on the other side until golden brown and cooked through.

Serve with your chosen toppings.

Energy Eggs

Scrambled eggs are cheap to make and are rich in protein and healthy fats. They'll keep your energy levels soaring for hours, while the addition of iron-rich spinach will keep your body smiling from the inside out.

<u>1 serving</u>

2 free-range eggs

1 teaspoon chopped fresh chives, plus a little extra for serving

a splash of coconut milk or almond milk

1 teaspoon extra virgin olive oil

a handful of baby spinach leaves

2 handfuls of watercress, chopped

1/2 ripe avocado, peeled and chopped

1 large vine tomato, sliced

sea salt and black pepper

To serve (optional)

1 large or 2 small slices of buckwheat bread, toasted

40g (1 1/2 oz) smoked salmon

In a bowl, whisk together the eggs, chives and milk. Add salt and pepper to taste, then set aside.

Heat the oil in a small pan, rolling it around so that it covers the entire pan. Add the spinach and watercress and wilt for 2–3 minutes.

Pour in the eggs and allow them to cook for 1–2 minutes, then use a spatula to separate them. Keep scrambling and cooking the eggs for a further 2–3 minutes, or until cooked to your liking.

Serve the scrambled egg, avocado and tomato on toast with the smoked salmon, if liked, and sprinkle over a few extra chopped chives and a little salt, if desired.

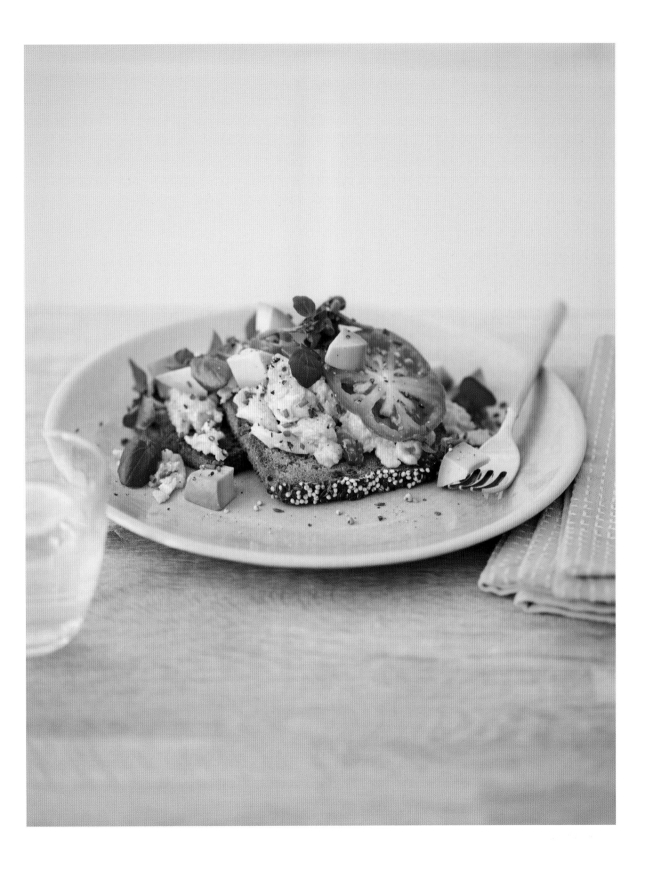

Vegetable Frittata & Speedy Salad

I love eating eggs daily, as they're high in hormone-healthy fats. My super-speedy salad makes a tasty and versatile side, too. The delicious addition of creamy avocado also helps to keep the body topped up with healthy fats.

2 servings

2 tablespoons coconut oil

1 small red onion, thinly sliced

1 red pepper, deseeded and thinly sliced

1 medium carrot, thinly sliced

25g sun-dried tomatoes in oil, drained and roughly chopped

1 medium courgette, thinly sliced

3 large organic free-range eggs

1 tablespoon coconut milk or almond milk

1 teaspoon turmeric

1 teaspoon dried oregano

1 large tomato, sliced

sea salt and freshly ground black pepper

For the speedy salad

2 handfuls of rocket

1/2 red onion, peeled and chopped

1/2 ripe avocado, peeled and chopped

10 cherry tomatoes, halved

extra virgin olive oil

balsamic vinegar

sea salt and black pepper

Heat the oil in a 20cm (8 inch) ovenproof omelette pan. Add the onion and cook gently until softened and golden brown.

Add the red pepper, carrot, sun-dried tomatoes and courgette, and cook for 3–4 minutes until softened.

Whisk together the eggs, milk and spices and season with salt and pepper. Pour the mixture into the pan and cook gently for 8–10 minutes, or until the frittata is browned underneath and almost set.

Meanwhile, make the salad. Put the rocket, onion, avocado and cherry tomatoes into a salad bowl and toss with a drizzle of olive oil and balsamic vinegar.

Remove the frittata from the hob and lay the sliced tomato on top. Place under a medium grill for 3–4 minutes, or until set on top and lightly browned.

Sprinkle the rocket salad with salt and pepper and serve with the frittata, cut into wedges.

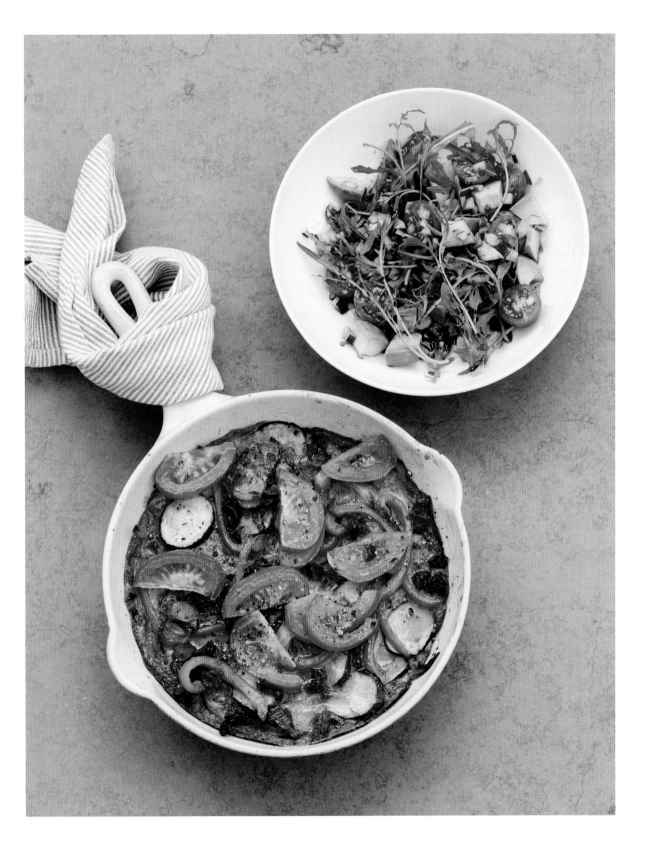

Thai Mango Salad

*Magical mango is hard to resist; however, don't save it for sweet dishes alone.
I incorporate it into all sorts of recipes – it works a treat in salsas and salads,
such as this one.*

<u>2 servings</u>

For the salad

150g (5$\frac{1}{2}$oz) mixed lettuce leaves,
   roughly torn

2 carrots, grated

a bunch of spring onions, finely sliced

1 red pepper, deseeded and sliced

100g (3$\frac{1}{2}$oz) beansprouts

1 fresh mild red chilli, deseeded and
   finely diced

70g (2$\frac{1}{2}$oz) mixed nuts, chopped

1 ripe mango, peeled and cut into 1cm
   ($\frac{1}{2}$ inch) cubes

salt and pepper

For the dressing

2 tablespoons extra virgin olive oil

juice of 1$\frac{1}{2}$ limes

2 tablespoons tamari

$\frac{1}{2}$ fresh red chilli, deseeded and chopped

1 teaspoon raw honey (optional)

a pinch of sea salt and cracked black pepper

a small handful of fresh coriander

Put all the salad ingredients into a large
salad bowl and toss together well.

In a blender, blitz together the dressing
ingredients until smooth, then drizzle
over the salad and serve with a sprinkling
of sea salt and cracked black pepper.

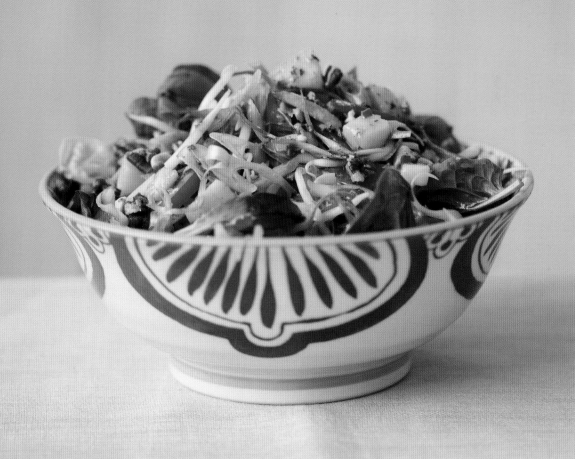

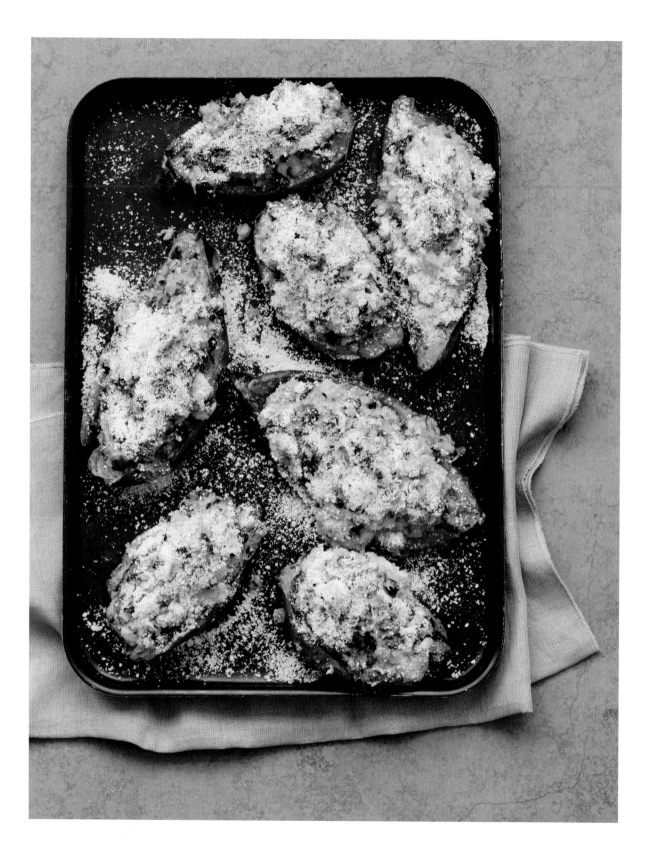

Stuffed Sweet Potato

Sweet potatoes are such a treat – naturally sweet, yet high in vitamins, minerals and a great source of healthy carbs. This nutritious dish is one of my favourite meals.

2 servings

2 large sweet potatoes, scrubbed clean

6 tablespoons coconut yogurt

2 tablespoons tahini

1 x 400g (14oz) BPA-free tin of black beans, drained and rinsed

1 ripe avocado, mashed

150g (5½oz) unsweetened sweetcorn, drained

2 ripe vine tomatoes, chopped

6–8 large slices of jalapeño chilli (fresh or from a jar), chopped

4 spring onions, chopped

2 small handfuls of fresh coriander, roughly chopped

2 garlic cloves, crushed (optional)

2 teaspoons turmeric

4 tablespoons ground almonds

salt and black pepper

steamed greens, to serve (*see* pages 196 and 198)

Preheat the oven to 180°C/350°F/ gas mark 4. Line a baking tray with baking paper.

Place the sweet potatoes on the prepared tray and bake for 45 minutes, or until softened and cooked through. Once cooked, cut in half lengthways, scoop out the flesh and put into a bowl, leaving the sweet potato skins intact (top tip: it helps if you leave some sweet potato inside the skins to prevent them collapsing).

Mix the sweet potato flesh with the yogurt and tahini. Stir in the black beans and the remaining ingredients, apart from the ground almonds. Season to taste.

Spoon the filling back into the potato skins, sprinkle 1 tablespoon of ground almonds over each half and grill for a few minutes until golden.

Serve one sweet potato with your choice of steamed greens for dinner and pack the other away for lunch the next day.

Cauliflower, Beetroot & Chickpea Wraps

These are a feast for the eyes as well as the tastebuds – vibrant, fresh and full of colour, thanks to that wonderful beetroot, a tasty detoxifier for the liver. It's also full of vitamins, minerals and glutamine, to keep the digestive system happy and healthy.

2 servings

For the roasting mix

1 x 400g (14oz) BPA-free tin of chickpeas, drained and patted dry

1/2 head of cauliflower, cut into small florets

2 medium beetroots, scrubbed clean and cut into cubes

2 teaspoons ground cumin

1 teaspoon paprika (optional)

2 teaspoons turmeric

sea salt

2 teaspoons extra virgin olive oil

For the mint yogurt

200g (7oz) coconut yogurt

80g (2³/4oz) cucumber, finely chopped

2 tablespoons finely chopped fresh mint

juice of 1/2 lemon

1/2 teaspoon ground cumin

a pinch of cayenne pepper

a pinch of salt and pepper

For the wraps

4 small gluten-free corn wraps

1 large carrot, grated

Mixed Herb Salad, to serve (see page 191)

Preheat the oven to 200°C/400°F/gas mark 6. Line a baking tray with baking paper.

Place the chickpeas, cauliflower and beetroots in a large mixing bowl and toss with the remaining roasting mix ingredients. Tip on to the prepared tray and roast in the oven for 20–30 minutes, or until the chickpeas are crisp, turning them halfway through the cooking time.

In the meantime, make the mint yogurt. Mix all the ingredients together, seasoning to taste and adding more mint if desired.

To serve, spoon some of the mint yogurt over each wrap, then add the roasted chickpeas, cauliflower and beetroots and the grated carrot.

Serve with a Mixed Herb Salad.

Pack the other portion away for lunch the next day, but keep the wraps separate and assemble just before eating.

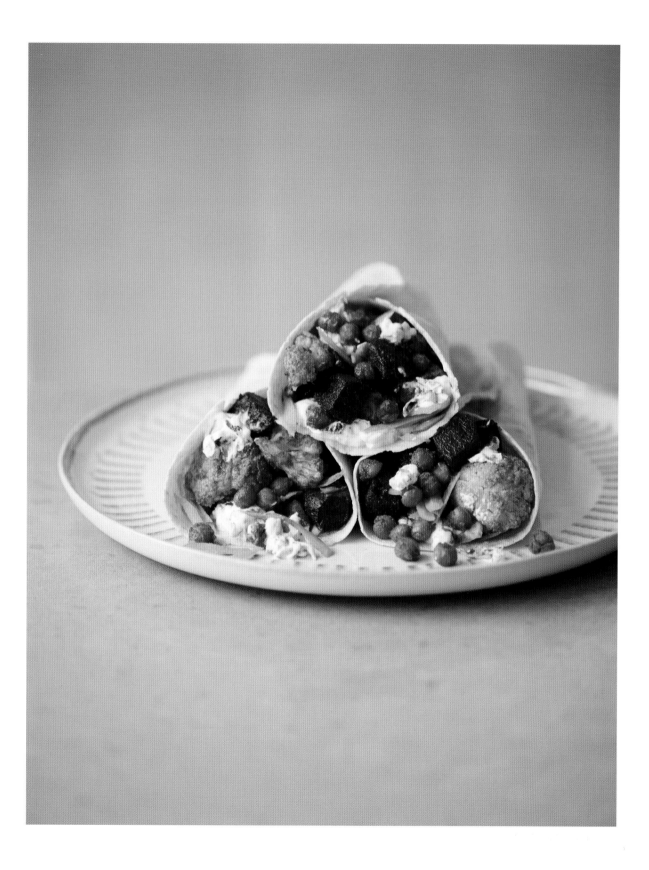

Lentil & Quinoa Sweet Potato Burgers

*Lentils are one of my favourite ingredients, as they're high in protein and iron –
both crucial for happy hormones. The addition of sweet potatoes and antioxidant-
rich carrots gives a touch of sweetness, making these burgers perfect for kids, too.*

2 servings

2 teaspoons extra virgin olive oil

1 large garlic clove, crushed

1 medium red onion, finely chopped

1/2 red pepper, finely chopped

1 medium carrot, grated

1 medium courgette, grated

100g (31/2oz) cooked lentils of your choice
(I prefer red or Puy)

50g (13/4oz) cooked quinoa

1 small sweet potato, steamed and lightly
mashed

15g (1/2oz) sunflower seeds

15g (1/2oz) pumpkin seeds

1 teaspoon chia seeds

1/2 teaspoon paprika

1/2 teaspoon ground cumin

1/2 teaspoon turmeric

1 teaspoon salt

a good grind of black pepper

a pinch of cayenne pepper

To serve

4 handfuls of mixed greens such as asparagus,
courgette, broccoli or pak choi

juice of 1 lemon, mixed with 3 tablespoons
extra virgin olive oil

Heat 1 teaspoon of oil in a large frying
pan over a medium heat. Gently fry
the garlic, stirring often, for about
1 minute. Add the onion and fry until
softened. Add the red pepper, carrot
and courgette and cook for a further
5 minutes until softened.

Transfer to a large bowl and stir in the
lentils, quinoa, mashed sweet potato,
sunflower, pumpkin and chia seeds,
spices, salt and pepper. Mix well, tasting
and adjusting the seasoning if needed.

Using your hands, shape the mixture into
4 patties, then place in the fridge to chill
for 10–15 minutes.

Heat a non-stick frying pan on a medium
heat for about 1 minute, then add
1 teaspoon of oil and heat slightly. Add
the burgers and cook for about 6–8
minutes on each side until browned and
cooked through.

Meanwhile, steam your choice of
mixed greens.

Drain the steamed vegetables and
serve them on a warm plate along with
2 burgers, drizzling with the lemon and
olive oil. Pack the other portion away for
lunch the next day.

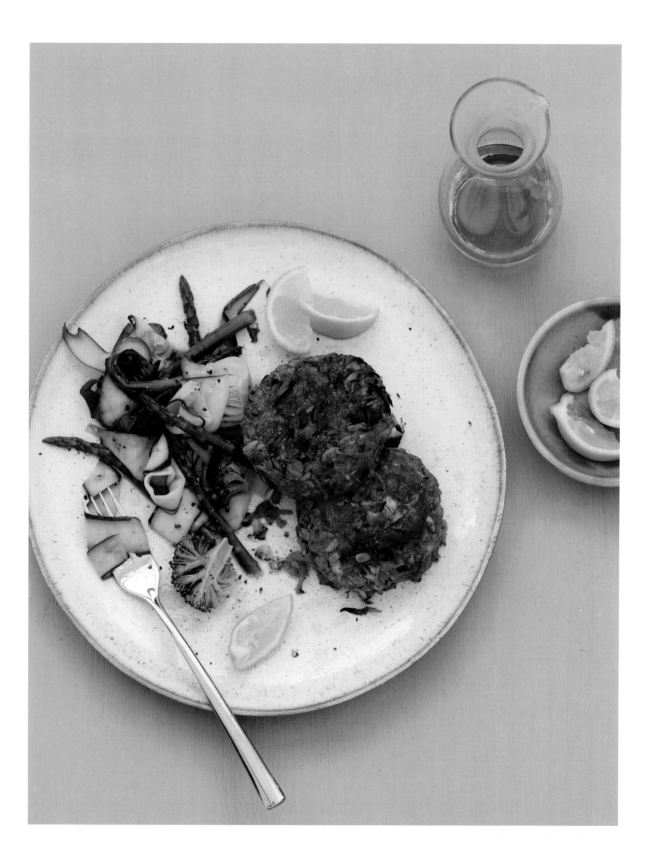

Pesto & Almond-crumbed Cod with Minty Peas

Cod is a good source of lean protein, and tastes delicious when paired with this pesto. Squeeze over plenty of fresh lemon juice for a taste of the Mediterranean and serve with my spin on mushy peas, with mint for healthy digestion.

2 servings

3½ tablespoons fresh pesto (*see* page 199)
3½ tablespoons ground almonds
extra virgin olive oil (optional)
320g (11½oz) skinless cod fillets
juice of ½ lemon
½ lemon, thinly sliced
a handful of cherry tomatoes, sliced in half
sea salt and cracked black pepper
Speedy Salad, to serve (*see* page 130)

For the minty peas

a drizzle of extra virgin olive oil
200g (7oz) frozen peas
2 spring onions, finely sliced
a small handful of fresh mint leaves, chopped
1 tablespoon coconut yogurt
a squeeze of fresh lemon juice
sea salt and cracked black pepper

Preheat the oven to 180°C/350°F/ gas mark 4. Line a baking tray with baking paper.

In a bowl, mix together the pesto and ground almonds until well combined, adding a drizzle of oil, if needed.

Place the cod fillets on the prepared tray, then spoon the pesto over each one, smoothing it over to cover the fish and pressing down with the back of a spoon to ensure that there are no cracks.

Drizzle over the lemon juice, then sprinkle with salt and pepper and lay the lemon slices over the top. Scatter the cherry tomatoes around the cod, then bake for 10–15 minutes, or until the fish is opaque and flakes easily.

Meanwhile, make the minty peas. Heat a drizzle of oil in a pan, then add the peas and spring onions, stirring constantly until warmed through.

Tip into a food processor with the remaining ingredients and pulse to form a purée. Taste, and add more mint, seasoning or lemon, if you like.

Serve the cod with the minty peas, and a Speedy Salad.

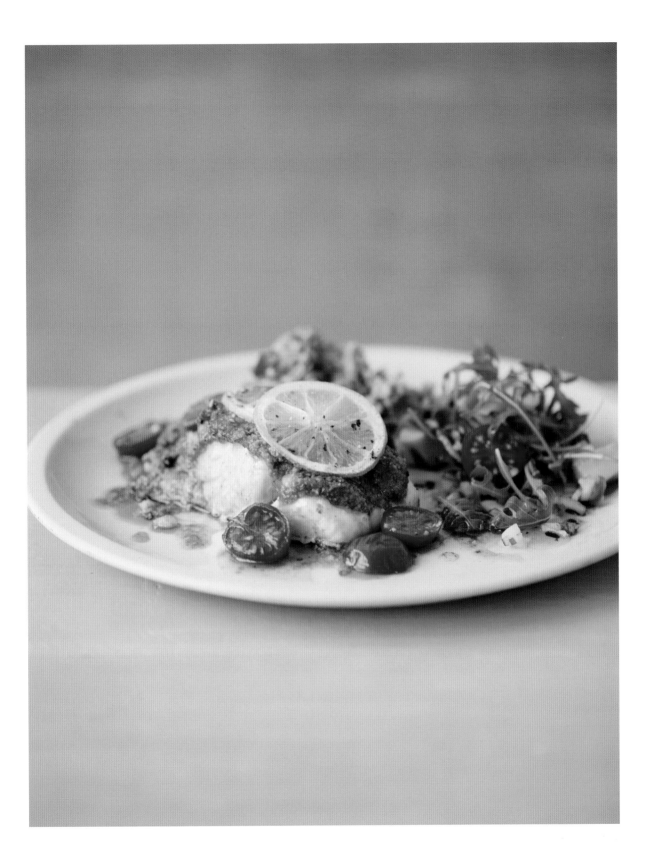

Flaked Salmon Sandwich

The wonderful protein and good fats in this simple meal will help to keep you feeling full for longer and alert for the rest of the day.

<u>1 serving</u>

1 leftover grilled salmon fillet

a small handful of rocket

1 teaspoon extra virgin olive oil

juice of 1/2 lemon

a pinch of sea salt and black pepper

1/2 avocado, mashed

2 slices of buckwheat bread

1/2 large vine tomato, sliced

1 tablespoon chopped fresh dill

1 tablespoon mixed seeds

1 serving of Purple Coleslaw (*see* page 195)

Use a fork to gently separate the salmon into flakes. It should have a torn look once you have finished. Set aside.

Toss the rocket in the oil and lemon juice and season with salt and pepper to taste. Set aside.

Spread the mashed avocado on the bread and lay the tomato slices on top.

Lay the rocket on top of the tomato slices. Season with salt and pepper.

Place the flaked salmon on top of the rocket and sprinkle with the dill and mixed seeds. Add one serving of purple slaw (store in a separate container if keeping in a lunchbox).

Before eating, add an extra squeeze of lemon juice, if you like, and enjoy.

Vegetarian Pad Thai

I love the exotic flavours of pad Thai, and anything with peanut butter will usually get my vote. This is my healthy vegan take on the exotic dish, and uses tempeh – fermented soybeans – as a source of plant-based protein.

<u>2 servings</u>

3 tablespoons coconut oil

200g (7oz) tempeh, cubed

125g (4¹/₂oz) flat brown rice noodles

juice of 1¹/₂ limes

3¹/₂ tablespoons tamari

3¹/₂ tablespoons crunchy sugar-free peanut butter

1 teaspoon dried chilli flakes

5 spring onions, finely sliced

1 garlic clove, finely chopped

2cm (³/₄ inch) piece of fresh ginger, peeled and finely chopped

2 medium carrots, cut into matchsticks

1 small head of broccoli, cut into florets

1 large red pepper, cut into thin strips

1 head of pak choi, chopped

100g (3¹/₂oz) sugar snap peas, chopped

1 small handful of fresh coriander leaves, roughly chopped

4 fresh basil leaves, roughly chopped

salt and freshly ground black pepper

To serve

2 tablespoons chopped salted peanuts

1 fresh long red chilli, deseeded and finely sliced

Heat half the coconut oil in a frying pan over a medium–high heat. Add the tempeh, seasoning with salt and pepper to taste. Cook until golden, then drain on kitchen paper and set aside.

Cook the noodles according to the packet directions. Drain well, then set aside.

Meanwhile, mix together the lime juice, tamari, peanut butter and chilli flakes in a small bowl, and set aside.

Heat the remaining coconut oil in a large frying pan. Add the spring onions, garlic and ginger and cook for 1 minute on a medium heat until fragrant.

Tip in the carrots, broccoli, red pepper, pak choi and sugar snaps and cook for about 3 minutes, or until the broccoli becomes vibrant green.

Stir in the lime mixture, tempeh and noodles and cook for 2–3 minutes, or until the noodles are heated through. Remove from the heat and stir in the coriander and basil.

Divide the pad Thai into two portions, serving one for dinner and packing the other away for the next day.

Serve scattered with chopped peanuts and fresh chilli.

Grilled Salmon with Broad Bean & Pesto Mash

This flavoursome, simple salmon dish is the perfect midweek meal, packed with heart-healthy fats and omega-3s, too. Silky broad beans are a great source of plant-based protein, and this mash works brilliantly with all sorts of mains.

2 servings

3 tablespoons extra virgin olive oil
juice of 2 lemons
zest of 1 lemon
2 garlic cloves, crushed
2 x 140g (5oz) salmon fillets
sea salt and cracked black pepper
steamed greens, to serve (*see* pages 196 and 198)

For the broad bean & pesto mash
200g (7oz) frozen baby broad beans
2 spring onions, finely chopped
a handful of fresh basil leaves
1 tablespoon coconut yogurt
juice of 1/2 lemon
2–3 tablespoons pesto (*see* page 199)

In a small bowl, mix together the oil, lemon juice, lemon zest, garlic and some salt and pepper to make a marinade.

Place the salmon fillets in a flat glass container and pour over the marinade, turning the fillets over so they are well coated. Cover the bowl and leave to marinate in the fridge for 20–30 minutes, if you have time.

Preheat the grill to medium or hot for 10–15 minutes. While waiting for it to heat up, start making the broad bean mash. Place the beans, spring onions and basil leaves in a large saucepan with a splash of water. Cover with a lid and steam for a few minutes, over a medium–low heat until softened and cooked.

Place in a blender with the remaining ingredients, adding the pesto to taste, and blend to your desired texture, adding sea salt and black pepper to taste. Set aside and keep warm.

Once the grill is hot, place the salmon fillets on a baking tray and brush with the excess marinade. Season with salt and pepper and grill for 6–8 minutes on each side, brushing the marinade over the fillets each time you turn them.

Serve one fillet of salmon on a bed of mash alongside your choice of steamed greens and pack the other portion away for lunch the next day.

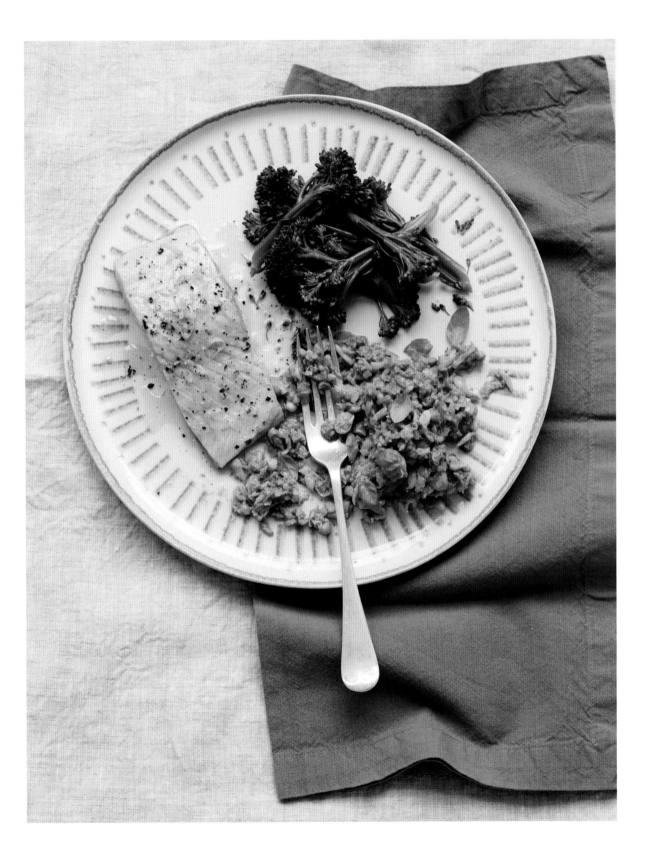

Pan-roasted Halibut with Artichokes & Broccoli

Firm, meaty halibut works well with all sorts of flavours. I love roasting it in one pan with two detoxifying wonders for the perfect hormone-balanced dish.

2 servings

300g (10½oz) tenderstem broccoli
360g (12¼oz) halibut fillets
2 tablespoons capers
1 lemon, thinly sliced
a handful of fresh parsley, finely chopped
1 tablespoon finely chopped fresh tarragon
1 tablespoon finely chopped fresh chives
Mixed Herb Salad or Cauliflower Mash, to serve
   (*see* pages 191 and 150)

For the artichokes

1 x 400g (14oz) BPA-free tin of artichoke
   hearts, drained and halved
2 garlic cloves, crushed
extra virgin olive oil
juice of 1 lemon
salt and pepper

Preheat the oven to 200°C/400°F/gas mark 6.

Arrange the artichokes in an ovenproof pan with the garlic. Drizzle over a splash of oil, a squeeze of lemon juice and season with salt and pepper. Bake for 10 minutes.

Remove the pan from the oven, add the broccoli and halibut fillets and scatter the capers into the pan. Season well, then lay the lemon slices over the halibut and drizzle everything with a splash of oil.

Spoon any juices over the fish and broccoli before returning the pan to the oven. Bake for a further 15 minutes, or until the fish is opaque and cooked through.

Before serving, sprinkle over the parsley, tarragon and chives.

Serve with a Mixed Herb Salad or some Cauliflower Mash.

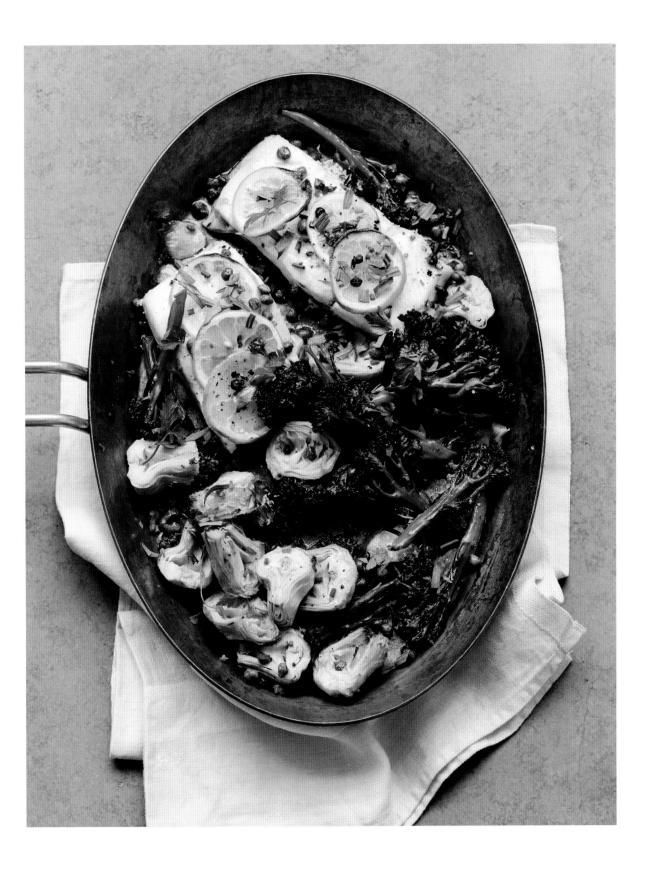

Sea Bass Parcels with Dill & Capers

Sea bass is one of my favourite sources of lean protein. It gets a health-kick here thanks to lemon, greens and tomatoes, which are high in vitamin C.

<u>2 servings</u>

2 sea bass fillets
juice of ½ lemon
2 tablespoons finely chopped fresh dill
1 tablespoon capers
½ lemon, thinly sliced
4 large vine-ripened tomatoes, sliced
sea salt and cracked black pepper

To serve
Minty Peas (*see* page 140)
steamed greens (*see* pages 196 and 198)

Preheat the oven to 180°C/350°F/gas mark 4. Place 2 pieces of baking paper on a baking tray.

Put each sea bass fillet on a piece of baking paper and drizzle over the lemon juice. Sprinkle over the dill and capers, then lay the lemon slices on top of each fillet. Place the tomato slices around the fish, then wrap each one into a parcel. Bake for 12–15 minutes, or until the fish is white and flakes easily.

Serve the sea bass parcels with Minty Peas and your choice of steamed greens.

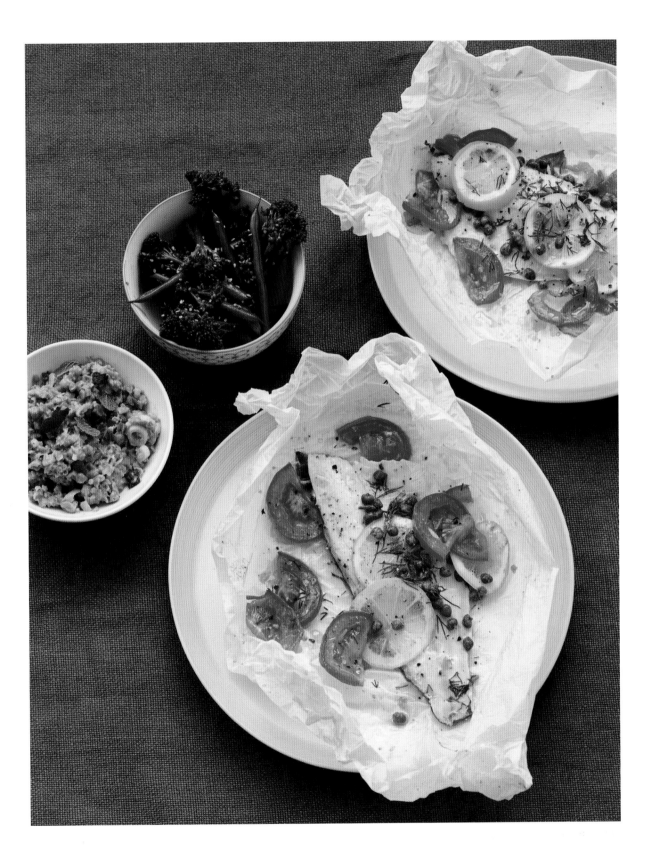

Lemon & Dill Salmon with Cauliflower Mash

Lemon and dill are such a classic combination with fish – and for good reason. Cauliflower can be whipped up into the most delicious mash replacement imaginable. Handily, cauliflower is also great at balancing out those hormones.

2 servings

3 tablespoons extra virgin olive oil
juice of 3 lemons
zest of 1 lemon
2 teaspoons finely chopped fresh dill
2 garlic cloves, crushed
2 x 150g (5½oz) salmon fillets
salt and black pepper

For the cauliflower mash
1 small head of cauliflower, cut into florets
3 garlic cloves, crushed and finely chopped
1 teaspoon finely chopped fresh chives
1 teaspoon finely chopped fresh thyme
1 tablespoon almond milk
2–3 tablespoons nutritional yeast (optional)
rock salt and cracked black pepper, to taste
1 teaspoon coconut oil or ghee (optional)

To serve
Speedy Salad (*see* page 130)

In a small bowl, mix together the oil, lemon juice, lemon zest, dill and garlic with some salt and pepper to make a marinade.

Place the salmon fillets in a flat glass container and pour over the marinade, turning the fillets over so they are well coated. Cover the bowl and leave the fillets to marinate in the fridge for 20–30 minutes, if you have time.

Meanwhile, make the salad and prep the mash.

Preheat the grill to medium–hot for 10–15 minutes. Meanwhile, start making the cauliflower mash. In a steamer, cook the cauliflower florets until tender. Alternatively, if you don't have a steamer, boil them in hot water until softened. Drain and pat dry.

Place the cauliflower in a food processor with all the remaining mash ingredients, apart from the oil, and blend until smooth and creamy. Season to taste and keep warm.

Once the grill is hot, place the salmon fillets on a baking tray and brush them with the excess marinade. Season with salt and pepper and grill for 6–8 minutes on each side, brushing the marinade over the fillets each time you turn them.

Serve one fillet of salmon on a bed of cauliflower mash alongside the salad and pack the other portion away for lunch the next day.

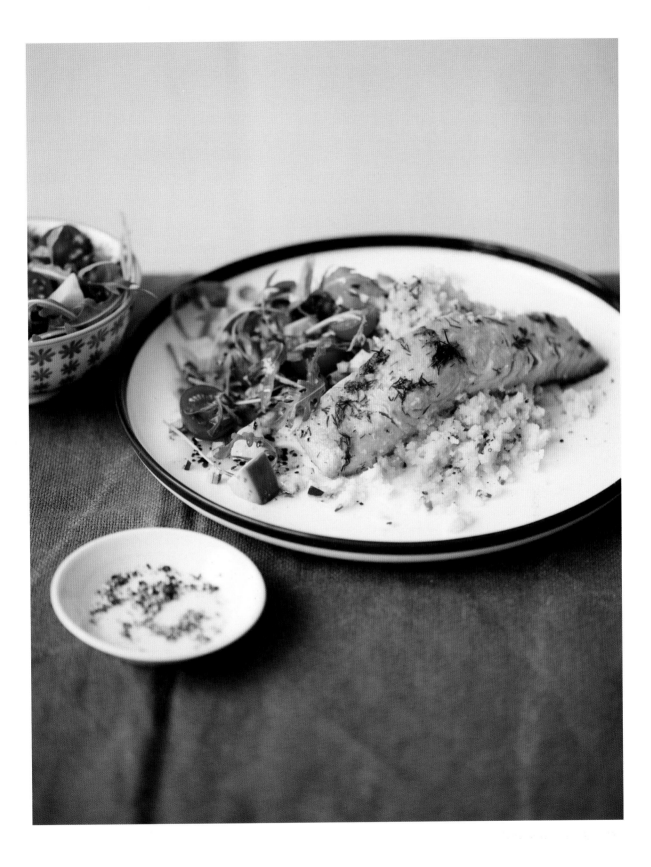

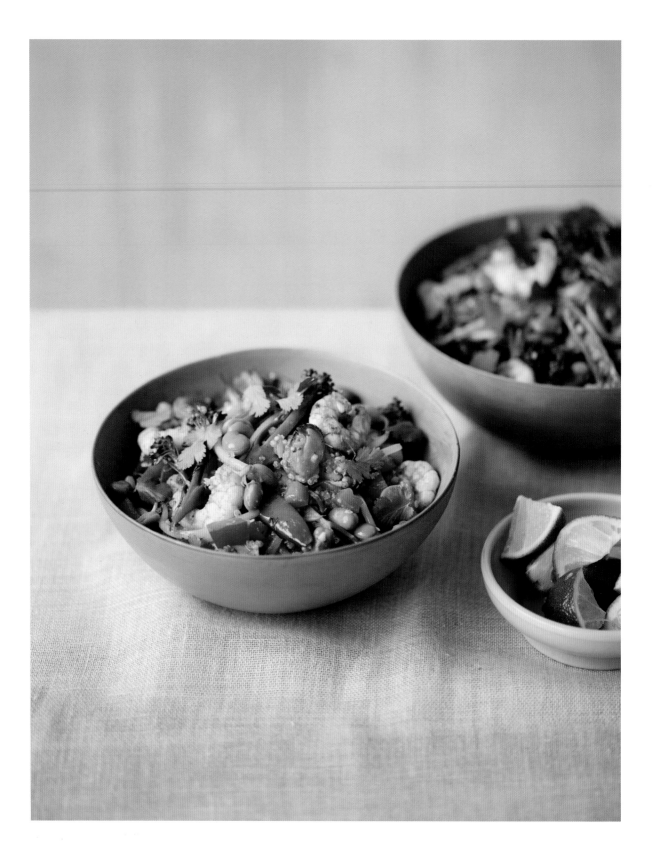

Thai-style Prawn & Mussel Stir-fry

Give your stir-fries a makeover with this Thai-inspired dish. I love the combination of citrus, spice and nuts in this stir-fry, which I like to serve alongside protein-boosting quinoa.

2 servings

For the paste

1 large fresh chilli, deseeded and finely chopped

a large handful of fresh coriander leaves, shredded

2 garlic cloves, crushed

2 teaspoons minced ginger

1 teaspoon raw honey

juice of 1 lime

For the stir-fry

100g (3^{1}/$_{2}$oz) prawns

100g (3^{1}/$_{2}$oz) mussels, shells removed

sesame seed oil

4 spring onions, finely chopped, or 1 shallot, chopped

70g (2^{1}/$_{2}$oz) broad beans or edamame beans

100g (3^{1}/$_{2}$oz) beansprouts

a handful of tenderstem broccoli, chopped

a handful of sugar snap peas, halved

2 red peppers, thinly sliced and chopped

1 tablespoon tamari

2 tablespoons fish sauce (optional)

For the quinoa

175g (6oz) cooked quinoa

To serve

a handful of fresh coriander leaves

2 tablespoons pumpkin seeds

juice of ^{1}/$_{2}$ lime

Start by making the paste by whizzing all the ingredients together in a small food processor until smooth.

Put the prawns and mussels into a bowl and pour over the paste, then cover and refrigerate for 1 hour if you have time. Prep the vegetables while you wait.

Heat some sesame seed oil in a large pan or wok, then add the spring onions and fry until lightly golden. Add the remaining vegetables and some seasoning and stir-fry until softened. Stir in the tamari.

Tip in the mussels and prawns, along with the fish sauce, if using, stirring well to combine. Toss and stir-fry for about 2 minutes, or until the seafood is cooked through, then remove from the heat and tip into a large bowl.

Stir the cooked quinoa into the stir-fry, then divide into two portions, one for this evening and the other to pack away ready for lunch the next day.

Sprinkle the coriander leaves and pumpkin seeds over both portions and drizzle over the lime juice.

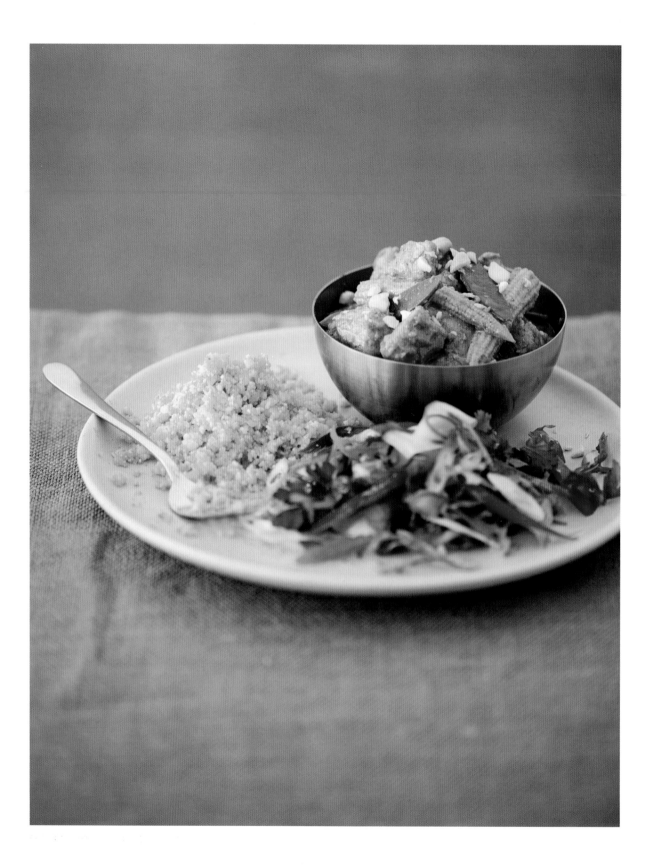

Satay-style Chicken with Cauliflower Rice

Almond butter is one of my store-cupboard essentials. It contains healthy fats and magnesium for energy, healthy bones and fibre, as well as skin-loving vitamin E. Cauliflower rice brings a host of additional phytonutrients and is ready in minutes.

2 servings

For the curry paste

3 red chillies, deseeded and chopped

4 teaspoons ground coriander

2 teaspoons ground cumin

4 stems of lemongrass, chopped

2 teaspoons minced ginger

3 shallots, chopped

6 garlic cloves, minced

zest and juice of 2 limes

1 tablespoon paprika

1 tablespoon extra virgin olive oil

For the chicken

1 tablespoon coconut oil

2 garlic cloves, minced

1 onion, finely chopped

300g (10½oz) skinless chicken breasts, diced

1 teaspoon chilli powder (optional)

85g (3oz) smooth almond butter

3–4 tablespoons curry paste (*see above*)

300ml (10fl oz) coconut milk

100g (3½oz) baby corn

100g (3½oz) mangetout

juice of 1 lime

50g (1¾oz) roughly chopped cashews

1 serving of Mixed Herb Salad (*see page 191*)

For the cauliflower rice

1 cauliflower, chopped

100ml (3½fl oz) vegetable stock

1 teaspoon ground turmeric

1 teaspoon ground cumin

sea salt and pepper

Put all the curry paste ingredients into a blender. Whizz to a smooth paste, adding a little water if needed.

Heat the coconut oil in a large pan. Add the garlic and onion. Cook for 2 minutes until the onions are slightly translucent.

Add the chicken and cook gently to seal the meat on all sides. Season with salt and add the chilli powder, if using.

Stir in the almond butter and curry paste until well coated. Add the coconut milk, baby corn, mangetout and 3–4 tablespoons water. Simmer for about 20 minutes.

Meanwhile, make the cauliflower rice. In small batches, pulse the cauliflower in a blender or food processor to a rice-like texture. Put into a saucepan with the stock and spices, cover and steam for 5–6 minutes. The cauliflower should be tender and fluffy but not too soft. Drain, stir through with a fork and keep warm.

When the chicken is cooked, add the lime juice and most of the cashews, and cook for a further 5 minutes.

Remove from the heat and sprinkle over the remaining cashew nuts. Serve one portion with some cauliflower rice and salad for dinner, and pack the other portion away for lunch the next day. Freeze any leftover curry paste for use another time.

Lemon & Rosemary Chicken

This baked lemon and rosemary chicken takes a classic and turns it into something special, thanks to the sweetness of alkalizing fresh lemon.

<u>2 servings</u>

1½ tablespoons extra virgin olive oil

300g (10½oz) boneless, skinless organic chicken breasts

1 medium sweet potato, washed and sliced

200ml (7fl oz) chicken broth or organic Chicken Stock (*see* page 166)

4 tablespoons lemon juice

½ tablespoon lemon zest

2 garlic cloves, minced

1 teaspoon crushed or ground fresh rosemary

¾ teaspoon dried thyme

a pinch of rock salt

a pinch of cracked black pepper

1 bay leaf

1 serving of Purple Coleslaw (*see* page 195)

sesame seeds

To garnish

2 sprigs of fresh rosemary

½ lemon, sliced

Preheat the oven to 200°C/400°F/gas mark 6.

Gently heat the oil in a large frying pan over a medium–high heat. Add the chicken and cook for 3 minutes on each side, or just until browned. Transfer the chicken to a large casserole dish and add the sweet potato.

In a small bowl, whisk together the chicken broth, lemon juice, lemon zest, garlic, rosemary, thyme, salt and pepper. Add the bay leaf.

Pour the lemon sauce over the chicken, then bake for 20–30 minutes, or until the chicken is cooked through and its juices run clear. Every 5–10 minutes, spoon the sauce from the dish over the chicken.

Divide the chicken and sweet potato into two portions. Garnish with fresh rosemary and lemon slices and serve one portion with purple slaw and a sprinkle of sesame seeds for dinner. Pack the other portion away ready for lunch the next day.

Chicken Salad

I'm always looking for new ways to use up leftovers. This salad is a great way to make the most of your roast: it's full of lean protein and healthy fats, while the pumpkin seeds provide lots of minerals to boost balance and hormone health.

<u>1 serving</u>

1 large vine tomato, chopped

3 spring onions, chopped

1 small baby gem lettuce, chopped

1 red pepper, deseeded and sliced

½ ripe avocado, peeled and cut into cubes

1 leftover Lemon & Rosemary Chicken breast (*see* opposite) or 200g (7oz) leftover Slow-cooked Roast Chicken (*see* page 178)

1 tablespoon pumpkin seeds

1 tablespoon sunflower seeds

1 serving of Purple Coleslaw (*see* page 195)

For the dressing

2 tablespoons extra virgin olive oil

4 tablespoons red wine vinegar or balsamic vinegar

1 teaspoon Dijon mustard

Put all the dressing ingredients into a glass jar and shake until well combined.

In a salad bowl, gently toss together the tomato, spring onions, lettuce, red pepper and avocado.

Tear the leftover chicken into bite-size pieces. Add to the salad bowl, along with the seeds, and mix until combined.

Pour the dressing over the salad and toss well to combine.

Store the salad and one serving of purple slaw in separate sealed containers in the fridge for lunch the next day.

Turkey Meatballs & Butternut 'Spaghetti'

This is comfort food at its finest. Herby meatballs served up with a rich, hearty tomato sauce, tossed with butternut 'spaghetti'. Simple, healthy and utterly delicious.

<u>2 servings</u>

For the meatballs

500g (1lb 2oz) turkey thigh mince
1 red onion, finely chopped
2 garlic cloves, minced
a handful of fresh parsley, finely chopped
6 fresh basil leaves, finely chopped
1 teaspoon Dijon mustard
1 1/2 teaspoons paprika
a pinch of cayenne pepper
2 tablespoons ground almonds
1 egg, beaten
sea salt and cracked black pepper
steamed greens, to serve (*see* pages 196 and 198)

For the sauce

1 teaspoon extra virgin olive oil
1 garlic clove, crushed and minced
1 red onion, finely chopped
1 red pepper, deseeded and chopped
1 courgette, finely chopped
1 x 400g (14oz) BPA-free tin of chopped tomatoes (the best quality you can afford)
5 large plum tomatoes, cut into quarters
2 teaspoons dried oregano
a handful of fresh basil leaves, plus extra to garnish
sea salt and cracked black pepper
juice of 1/2 lemon

For the butternut 'spaghetti'

2 teaspoons coconut oil
2 fresh sage leaves, finely chopped
1/2 large butternut squash, peeled and spiralized (you can buy this ready-made)

Using your hands, mix together all the meatball ingredients in a bowl, adding some seasoning. Shape into 10–12 meatballs, then place in the fridge to chill for 1 hour.

Meanwhile, make the sauce. Heat the oil in a saucepan on a medium heat. Gently fry the garlic, stirring often, for about 1 minute. Add the onion and fry until softened. Add the red pepper and courgette and fry for a further 5 minutes. Tip in the tomatoes, along with the oregano, basil and seasoning. Bring to a slight boil, then reduce the heat and simmer for about 15 minutes, until the sauce has thickened and the fresh tomatoes have started to soften. Using a spoon, squash the fresh tomatoes into the sauce, then stir in the lemon juice.

Tip the sauce into a roasting tin or casserole dish and set aside. Preheat the oven to 180°C/350°F/gas mark 4.

Heat a little more oil in a frying pan. Fry the meatballs for 1 minute or so on each side. Place them in the sauce, then bake, uncovered, for about 15 minutes, or until the meatballs are cooked through.

For the 'spaghetti', melt the coconut oil in a pan and gently fry the sage leaves until crisp. Stir in the squash, season and fry for 3–5 minutes to heat through.

Serve one portion with your choice of steamed greens or a side salad, if liked. Pack away the second portion for lunch the next day.

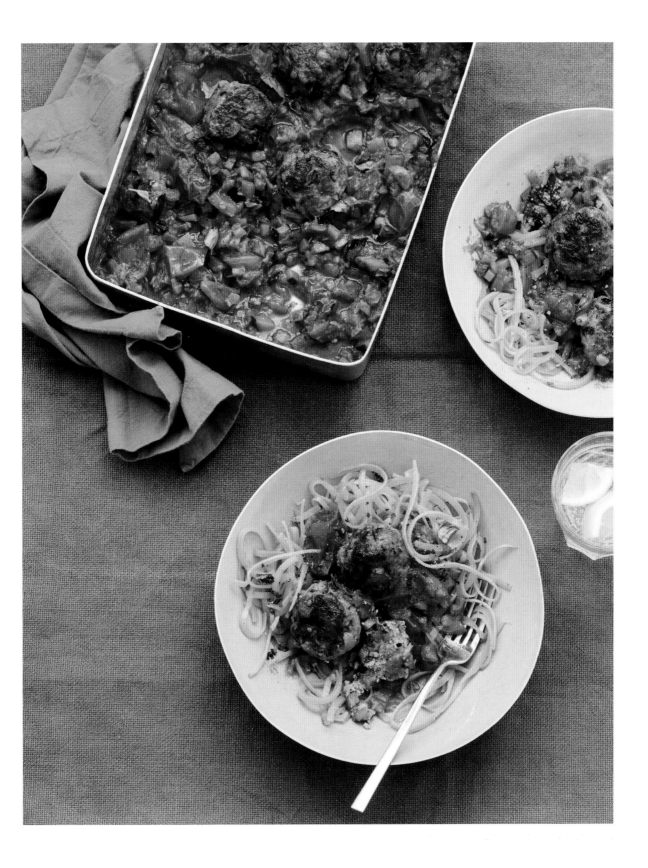

Cauliflower Pizza

Who said pizzas have to be unhealthy? Mixed with protein-rich quinoa flour and ground almonds, cauliflower creates a deliciously crisp base – all without gluten or added nasties. Perfect with tomato sauce and your favourite toppings.

<u>2 servings</u>

140g (5oz) cauliflower florets

100g (3½oz) quinoa flour or gluten-free flour

50g (1¾oz) ground almonds

¼ teaspoon bicarbonate of soda

½ teaspoon salt

1 teaspoon aluminium and gluten-free baking powder

¼ teaspoon paprika

1 egg white

2 tablespoons extra virgin olive oil

For the marinara sauce

½ tablespoon extra virgin olive oil

3 garlic cloves, crushed and minced

1 x 400g (14oz) BPA-free tin of chopped tomatoes (the best quality you can afford)

juice of ½ lemon

1 teaspoon dried oregano

4 fresh basil leaves, chopped

sea salt and cracked black pepper

Toppings

grilled and sliced chicken breast

sliced tomatoes

sliced red or yellow peppers

fresh basil leaves

Start by making the marinara sauce. Heat the oil in a pan, add the garlic and cook, stirring often, until golden. Add the remaining ingredients, seasoning to taste, and simmer uncovered on a low–medium heat until the sauce thickens. Stir often as the sauce can catch and burn easily.

Preheat the oven to 200°C/400°F/gas mark 6.

Place the cauliflower in a food processor and pulse until it resembles rice. Transfer to a mixing bowl and combine with the flour, ground almonds, bicarbonate of soda, salt, baking powder and paprika.

In a separate bowl, whisk together the egg white, oil and 50ml (2fl oz) of water.

Make a well in the middle of the flour mix, then pour in the egg white mixture. Mix well to form a dough, adding a splash more water if it feels dry.

Divide the pizza dough between two 25cm (10 inch) non-stick round baking trays, pressing down with the back of a spoon to ensure an even thickness. Bake for 20 minutes, or until golden. Flip the pizza bases over and return to the oven for a further 5 minutes to bake the underside, then turn out on to a cooling rack.

Once the pizza bases have cooled slightly, set one base aside. Spread the other base evenly with half the sauce, add your toppings, then return to the oven until golden brown and the toppings are cooked through.

Scatter the pizza with basil leaves and serve with a large mixed salad. Pack the remaining base away for topping and cooking the next day.

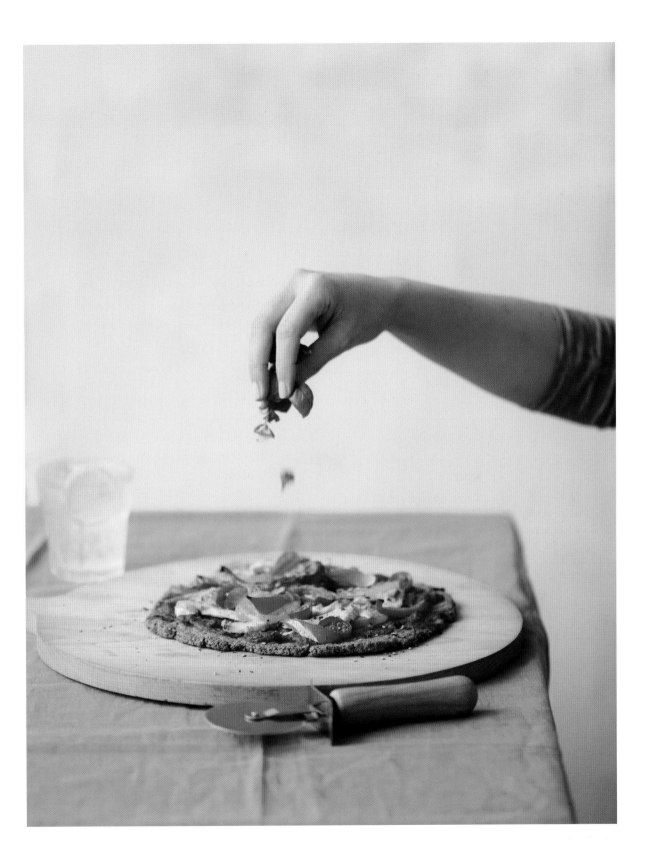

Chicken & Vegetable Stir-fry

I love stir-fries. This one is full of exotic tastes, and is a great source of fibre. Sesame seeds are a great addition, as they add texture and minerals, including manganese, calcium and magnesium.

2 servings

2 teaspoons unscented coconut oil

4 garlic cloves, crushed

1 red onion, diced

1 fresh red chilli, chopped

300g (10½oz) organic chicken breasts, diced

350ml (12fl oz) chicken stock

2 tablespoons gluten-free soy sauce or tamari

3 tablespoons sesame oil

2 spring onions, chopped

200g (7oz) pak choi, chopped

200g (7oz) mangetout

2 red peppers, sliced

1 small head of broccoli, chopped

5 water chestnuts, peeled and sliced

a handful of shiitake mushrooms

2 tablespoons sesame seeds, to garnish

sea salt and cracked black pepper

mixed salad, to serve (*see pages 191 and 192*)

Heat 1 teaspoon of coconut oil in a saucepan. Add half the garlic, half the onion, and the chilli. Stir over a medium heat until the aroma starts to rise.

Add the chicken pieces, stock and 1 tablespoon of soy sauce and stir-fry until cooked through. Season to taste.

Spoon the chicken into a separate bowl, reserving the stock for later use. Drizzle 1 tablespoon of sesame oil over the chicken, toss and set aside.

Put the remaining teaspoon of coconut oil into a large wok with the remaining garlic and red onion, and stir.

Add the spring onions, pak choi, mangetout, red peppers, broccoli, water chestnuts, shiitake mushrooms and the reserved chicken stock and stir-fry for 3–5 minutes, stirring continuously.

Add the remaining tablespoon of soy sauce, the 2 tablespoons of sesame oil and the reserved chicken pieces. Stir-fry for a further minute to heat through. Remove from the heat and sprinkle with the sesame seeds.

Divide the stir-fry into two portions. Serve one portion for dinner with your choice of salad. Pack the other portion away for lunch the next day.

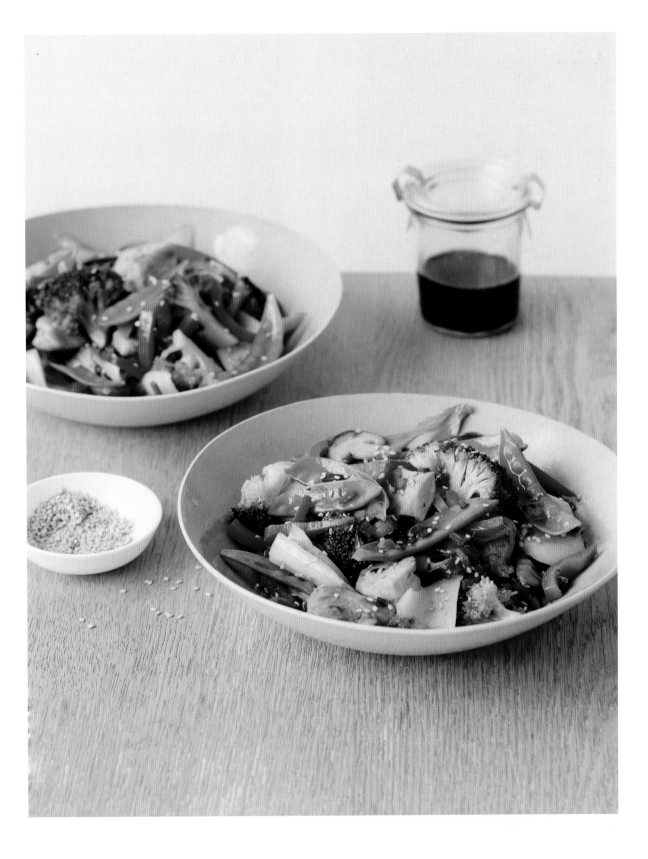

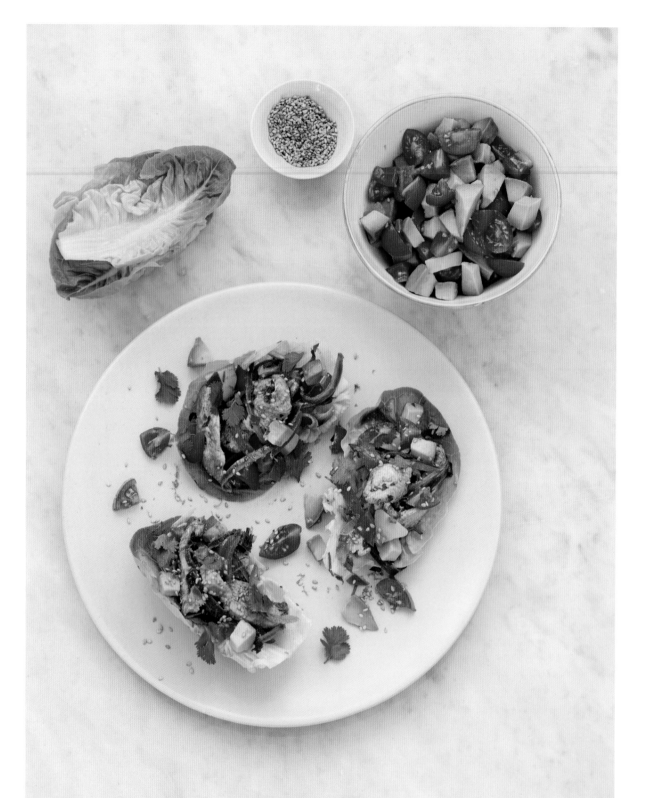

Chicken Fajita Wraps

Every household needs a Mexican night – and this is a brilliantly healthy way to enjoy classic fajitas. The avocado salsa is full of healthy fats, which can reduce inflammation and in turn help your body to absorb nutrients better.

2 servings

3 organic chicken breasts, cut into strips
1 teaspoon paprika
1 teaspoon ground cumin
1 teaspoon dried oregano
1 teaspoon coconut oil
4–6 tablespoons chicken stock
2 red onions, finely sliced
1 garlic clove, minced
1 red pepper, deseeded and sliced
1 green pepper, deseeded and sliced
a small handful of fresh coriander, finely chopped, plus a few extra leaves
a small handful of fresh flat-leaf parsley, finely chopped
juice and zest of 1 lime
2–3 baby gem lettuces, washed and leaves kept whole
1 tablespoon sesame seeds, to serve

For the avocado salsa

1 ripe avocado, peeled and chopped
10 cherry tomatoes, chopped
a squeeze of lime juice

In a bowl, mix together the chicken and spices, then set aside.

Heat the coconut oil in a pan, add the chicken strips with 1–2 tablespoons of chicken stock, and cook until browned all over. Remove using a slotted spoon and set aside. Tip the onions and garlic into the pan and cook until browned, adding a little more oil if needed.

Return the chicken to the pan, along with the red and green peppers and the remaining chicken stock, and stir-fry until the chicken is cooked through and the peppers have softened – add a few tablespoons of water if necessary to prevent sticking. Set aside to cool slightly.

Meanwhile, prepare the avocado salsa by mixing all the ingredients in a bowl.

When ready to serve, stir the chopped coriander, parsley, lime juice and zest into the chicken.

Add a spoonful of the chicken mixture on to each lettuce leaf, top with the avocado salsa and sprinkle with the sesame seeds and a few coriander leaves.

Remember to get your lunchbox ready for the next day – store the chicken, salsa and lettuce wraps separately in your lunchbox and assemble just before eating.

Chunky Chicken Soup

My chicken soup is food for the soul – hearty, comforting and incredibly satisfying.

3–4 servings

1 1/2 tablespoons extra virgin olive oil

3 garlic cloves, crushed

1 onion, finely diced

500–600g (1lb 2oz–1lb 5oz) leftover roast chicken, deboned

4 carrots, roughly chopped

1 leek, finely sliced

3 sticks of celery, roughly chopped

1/2 butternut squash, deseeded, peeled and diced

2 courgettes, roughly chopped

200ml (7fl oz) Chicken Stock (*see below*)

1 teaspoon salt

black pepper, to taste

3/4 teaspoon dried thyme

3/4 teaspoon dried rosemary

a good pinch of saffron

1 bay leaf

Chop Chop Salad, to serve (*see page 192*)

Heat the oil slightly in a large soup pot and brown the garlic and onion.

Add the remaining ingredients, then pour in 1 litre (1¾ pints) of water, making sure everything is covered. Bring to the boil over a high heat.

Skim off any foam that rises to the top, then turn the heat to low and simmer for 30–40 minutes, or until the vegetables are tender. Add more water as needed.

Once the soup is ready, dish up a hearty bowl for lunch and serve with a side of Chop Chop Salad, if liked.

Allow the rest of the soup to cool, then divide into portions and place in the freezer for later use.

Chicken Stock

Homemade stock is tastier and more nutritious than any shop-bought cube.

Makes 2 litres (3½ pints)

1 whole 1.3–1.8kg (3–4lb) organic chicken

1 teaspoon black peppercorns

1 bay leaf

3 sticks of celery, roughly chopped

1 large red onion, peeled and roughly chopped

3 large carrots, peeled and roughly chopped

2 red peppers, seeded and chopped

4 teaspoons apple cider vinegar

3 sprigs of fresh parsley

2 sprigs of fresh thyme

3 sprigs of fresh rosemary

1 sprig of fresh oregano

1 teaspoon coarse sea salt

Place everything in a large saucepan. Add cold water to cover and bring to a boil.

Skim off any foam from the surface, reduce the heat to low and simmer for 3–4 hours.

Once cooked, allow the stock to cool completely, then strain into a clean container/s discarding the solids and aromatics. Freeze for up to 6 months.

For vegetable stock, follow the same method but leave out the chicken and oregano. Use fresh tarragon in place of the rosemary and add 1 chopped leek and 3 crushed garlic gloves.

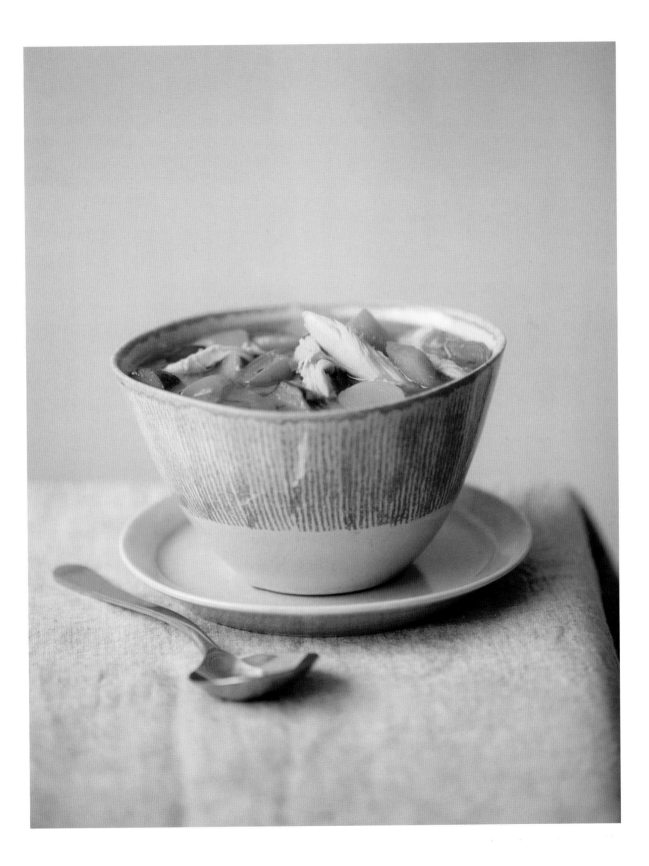

Zesty Turkey Pasta Salad

This dish is the perfect blend of fats, protein and carbs, and will help you to 'eat the rainbow'. Turkey is a wonderful source of lean protein – perfect for staving off hunger hormones and for building muscle, too.

2 servings

For the turkey

juice and zest of 1 lemon
1 garlic clove, crushed
1 teaspoon raw honey
1 tablespoon Dijon mustard
1/2 teaspoon salt
1 teaspoon cracked black pepper
300g (10 1/2 oz) turkey breast

For the salad

100g gluten-free pasta
2 handfuls of spinach
a handful of mixed leaves
1/4 cucumber, chopped
1 red pepper, chopped
1 carrot, grated
1 courgette, julienned
6 sun-dried tomatoes, chopped
a small bunch of fresh parsley, finely chopped
2 tablespoons pumpkin seeds

For the vinaigrette

3 1/2 tablespoons extra virgin olive oil
2 tablespoons red wine vinegar
1 tablespoon Dijon mustard
1 tablespoon lemon juice
1 garlic clove, crushed and minced
1/2 teaspoon dried oregano
salt and black pepper

To prepare the turkey, mix together the lemon juice and zest, garlic, honey, mustard, salt and pepper. Spoon this over the turkey, ensuring that it is completely coated, then cover and refrigerate for 1 hour to marinate, or longer if you have the time.

Once ready to cook, preheat the oven to 180°C/350°F/gas mark 4. Line a baking tray with greaseproof paper.

Place the marinated turkey on the prepared tray and cook for 18–20 minutes, or until cooked through.

Meanwhile, cook the pasta and allow it to cool slightly.

Toss together all the remaining salad ingredients in a large bowl and set aside.

Place all the vinaigrette ingredients in a glass jar with a lid and shake until well combined.

Once ready to serve, shred the turkey into strips and add to the salad bowl. Drizzle the vinaigrette over the salad and toss well. Serve one portion for dinner (hot or cold) and pack one portion away for lunch the next day.

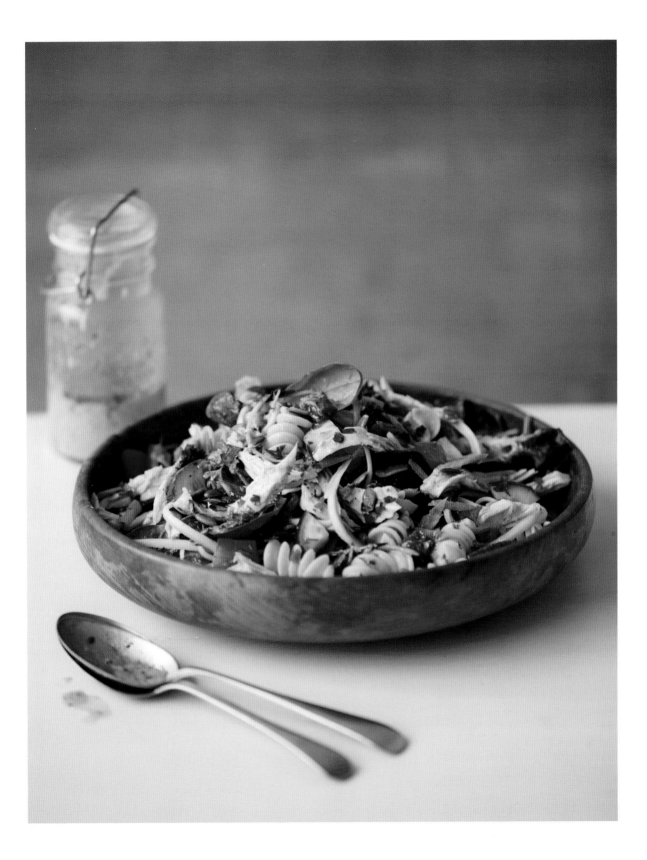

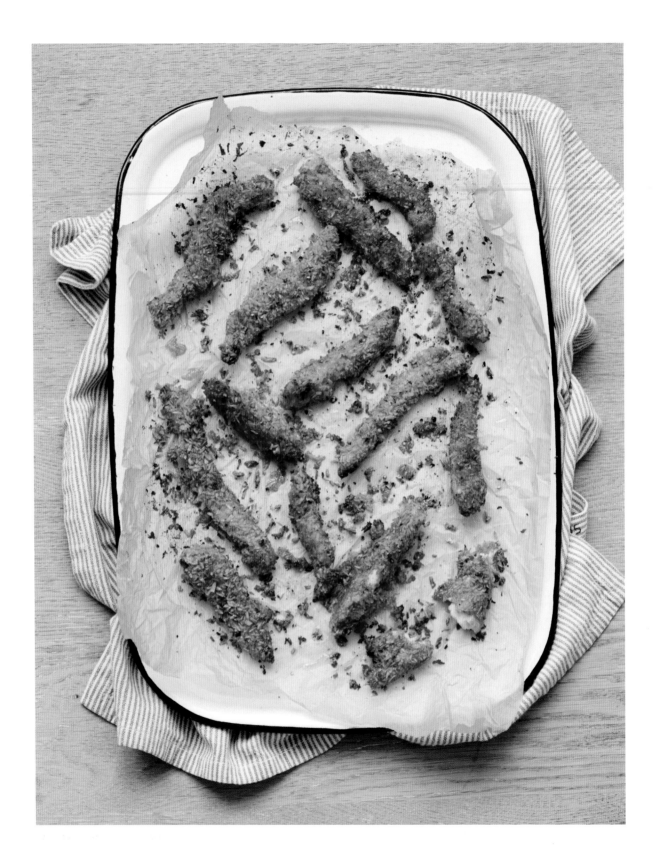

Coconut-crumbed Chicken

This is my tasty take on classic chicken goujons. The desiccated coconut adds crunch plus a good dose of body-loving fats. Dish them up with a simple sugar-free tomato ketchup, herby salad and sweet potato fries for an easy mid-week meal.

2 servings

1 large free-range egg

4 tablespoons coconut flour

6 tablespoons desiccated coconut

2 teaspoons paprika

1 garlic clove, minced

3/4 teaspoon rock salt

1 teaspoon cracked black pepper

300g (10 1/2 oz) organic free-range chicken breasts, cut into strips

To serve

Cauliflower Mash (*see* page 150)

Mixed Herb Salad (*see* page 191)

Preheat the oven to 180°C/350°F/ gas mark 4. Line a baking tray with baking paper.

Whisk the egg and set aside. Put the coconut flour into one bowl and the desiccated coconut into another.

Stir the paprika, garlic, salt and black pepper into the dessicated coconut until well combined.

Taking one chicken strip at a time, dunk it first into the coconut flour, then into the beaten egg, then into the desiccated coconut. Lay all the strips on the prepared tray. Sprinkle over more pepper, if you like, and bake for 18 minutes, or until the chicken is cooked through.

Divide into two portions. Serve one portion for dinner with Cauliflower Mash and Mixed Herb Salad, and pack the other portion away for lunch the next day.

Rich Lamb Curry

Who needs an expensive takeaway when curries are this simple and delicious to make at home? Turmeric is one of my favourite healing spices and lends this curry a lovely richness, along with anti-inflammatory properties – you can't go wrong.

2 servings

500g (1lb 2oz) lamb, diced

1 teaspoon aluminium and gluten-free baking powder

2 large onions, chopped

4 garlic cloves

15g (½oz) fresh coriander, chopped

3 fresh chillies, deseeded and chopped

2 tablespoons extra virgin olive oil

30g (1oz) fresh ginger

1 tablespoon coconut oil

1 tablespoon ground turmeric

1 tablespoon garam masala

3 tablespoons ground cumin

1 tablespoon ground coriander

1 tablespoon chilli powder

6–8 cardamom pods

5 large tomatoes, blanched and blended, or 400g (14oz) pure passata

500ml (18fl oz) hot lamb stock, or you can use vegetable or Chicken Stock (see page 166)

400ml (14fl oz) coconut milk

1 cinnamon stick

a large handful of kale

1 carrot, roughly chopped

100g (3½oz) mangetout

2 large handfuls of spinach

1 courgette, roughly chopped

sea salt and black pepper, to taste

Cauliflower Rice (see page 155), to serve

———————

Sprinkle the lamb with the baking powder and some pepper and refrigerate while you prepare the other ingredients.

In a blender, combine the onions, garlic, coriander, chillies, olive oil and ginger, adding up to 150ml (5fl oz) of water if you find it hard to blend.

Heat the coconut oil in a deep pan. Add the lamb and sauté until it is sealed. Remove the lamb with a slotted spoon and set aside. (You may need to seal the meat in batches.)

Pour the blended mixture into the same pan and simmer for 5 minutes, until any liquid has evaporated. Then add the spices and simmer for a further 5 minutes, stirring to prevent sticking.

Stir in the tomatoes and the stock. Simmer for a further 5 minutes, then stir in the coconut milk, add the cinnamon stick and return the lamb to the pan. Cover and simmer on a low heat for 1½ –2 hours, or until the lamb is tender.

Add the kale and carrot and simmer for 20 minutes. Stir occasionally to prevent sticking.

Add the mangetout, spinach and courgette and simmer for a further 5–8 minutes until the vegetables are tender.

Remove the lid and reduce on a high heat for 5–10 minutes if necessary, before removing the cinnamon stick and cardamom pods.

Serve one portion with the cauliflower rice and pack the other portion away for lunch the next day.

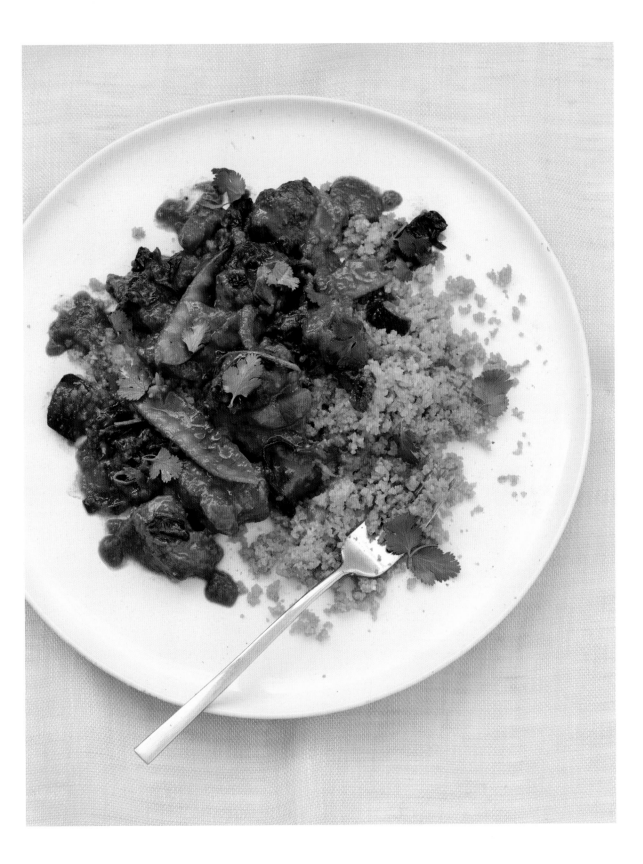

Slow-cooked Lamb & Roots

This is one of my favourite dishes to serve to friends and family: the lamb is meltingly tender and guaranteed to make you go back for seconds.

<u>4 servings</u>

1kg (2lb 4oz) lamb shoulder
3 garlic cloves, 1 quartered the rest crushed
2 tablespoons extra virgin olive oil
2 large carrots, chopped
2 large parsnips, chopped
1 onion, cut into quarters
1 large leek, trimmed and sliced
450ml (16fl oz) hot stock
3 sprigs of fresh rosemary
sea salt and cracked black pepper

To serve
Creamy Salad (*see* page 176)
steamed greens (*see* pages 196 and 198)

Preheat the oven to 180°C/350°F/ gas mark 4.

Prepare the lamb for seasoning. Drag the tip of a sharp knife in lines across the meat, creating shallow scores through the top layer of the lamb shoulder, cross-hatching the entire surface on both sides.

Drive the tip of the knife and twist it into the meat in four different areas, then stuff each hole with a quarter clove of garlic. The garlic should be completely buried in the lamb. Rub both sides of the lamb with oil and the crushed garlic and season with sea salt and black pepper.

Place the lamb in the centre of a medium to large deep roasting dish and lay the carrots, parsnips, onion and leek around it. Pour the stock over the vegetables on either side of the lamb, then place a sprig of rosemary on top of the meat and one on either side.

Cover the roasting tin with kitchen foil and roast for about 2–2½ hours. Then remove the foil and return to the oven for 30–40 minutes, or until cooked to your liking.

Meanwhile, start preparing your sides of choice.

Once the lamb is cooked, remove it from the oven and allow to stand for 30–40 minutes, then serve with the salad and greens. Remember to portion out enough lamb, salad and greens for lunch the next day.

Any additional leftovers can be used to make Lamb Wraps (*see* page 176) or can be frozen for later use.

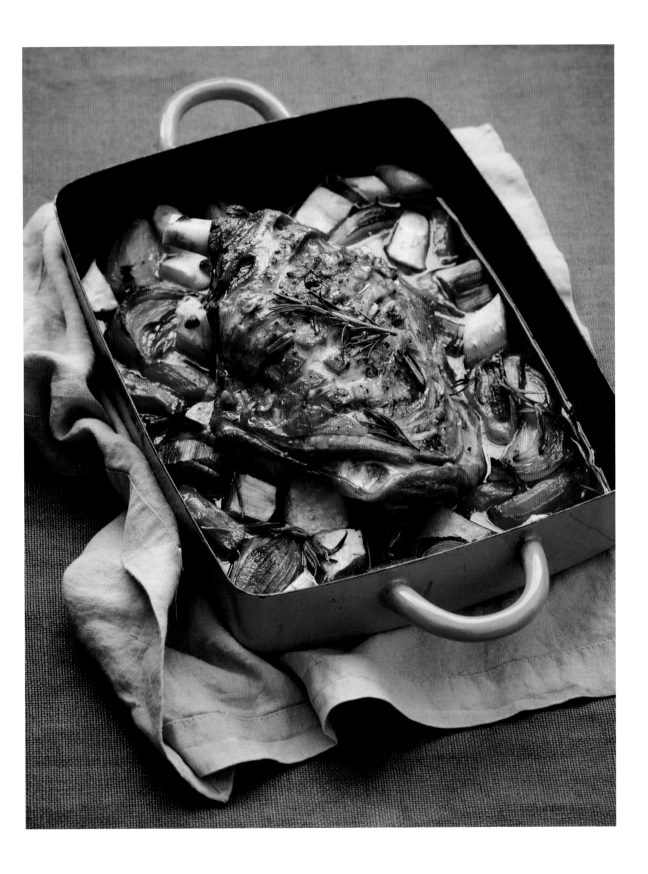

Lamb & Creamy Salad Wraps

This lamb wrap is full of flavour and will keep those blood sugars balanced, while the mixed salad will add some detoxifying goodness.

2 servings

120g (4¼oz) cooked lamb, sliced or shredded
4 gluten-free corn wraps (store-bought)
5 tablespoons creamy salad (*see* below)

For the salad

1 large head of Cos lettuce or other favourite lettuce, chopped
a small handful of watercress
½ cucumber, sliced
1 red pepper, deseeded and chopped
1 large carrot, grated
1 stick of celery, finely diced
a small handful of fresh flat-leaf parsley
50g (1¾oz) walnuts, roughly broken up
2 tablespoons sunflower seeds

For the creamy dressing

½ teaspoon Dijon mustard
2 tablespoons apple cider vinegar
2 tablespoons extra virgin olive oil
2 tablespoons raw tahini
1 teaspoon ground turmeric
½ teaspoon rock salt
cracked black pepper, to taste

Prepare the salad by combining the vegetables, parsley, walnuts and sunflower seeds in a bowl.

Blend all the dressing ingredients with 3 tablespoons of water, then drizzle over the salad and stir well to combine. Ideally, allow the salad to sit in the fridge for 30 minutes (it tastes better when you do this), though it will still be very tasty if you serve it right away.

To assemble, place the lamb and the creamy salad slightly off-centre on each wrap. Don't overfill. Fold in the sides so they nearly touch, then bring up the bottom of the wrap and start rolling.

In your lunchbox, you may want to keep the lamb, salad and wraps separate and assemble before eating, as otherwise they will become soggy.

Eat any leftover lamb and salad that don't make it into the wrap another time.

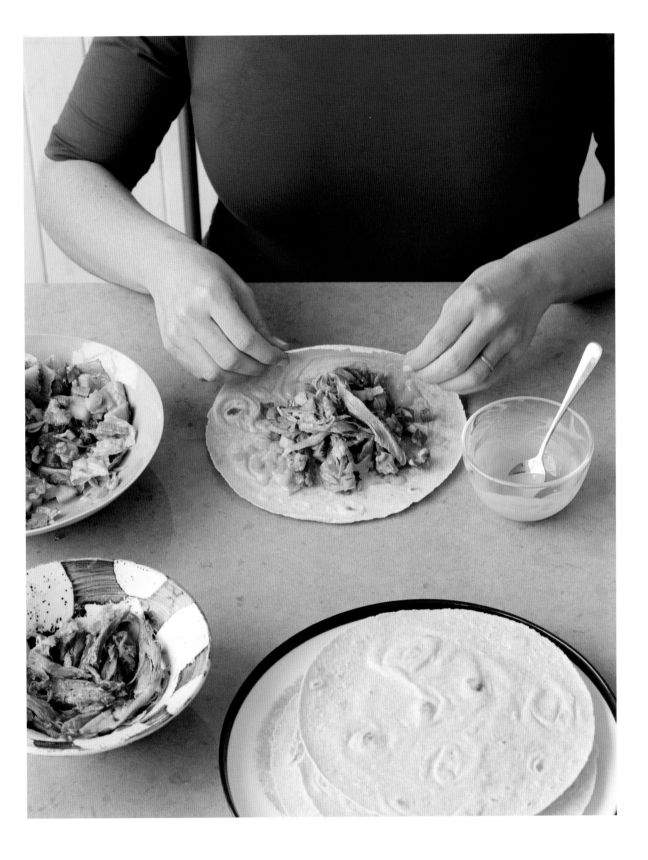

Slow-cooked Roast Chicken & Veg

Is there anything more delicious and heart-warming than a family roast on a Sunday afternoon? If possible, prepare the chicken the night before.

<u>4 servings</u>

1 whole free-range organic chicken (about 1.8kg/4lb)

extra virgin olive oil

1 bulb of garlic, separated into peeled cloves

2–3 large unwaxed lemons

25g (1oz) fresh thyme sprigs

25g (1oz) fresh rosemary sprigs

200g (7oz) carrots, cut into batons

200g (7oz) parsnips, cut into chunks

200ml (7fl oz) Chicken Stock (*see* page 166)

sea salt and cracked black pepper

Rainbow Salad, to serve (*see* page 192)

———————

Rub the chicken inside and out with a generous amount of salt and cracked black pepper. Cover tightly and refrigerate overnight.

In the morning, mix together 2 tablespoons of oil, 6 crushed garlic cloves and the juice of 1 lemon. Scoop the pulp out of the juiced lemon and set it aside.

Rub the oil mixture all over the chicken, spread the lemon pulp over the top of the chicken, cover tightly and place it back in the fridge for 1 hour.

Preheat the oven to 190°C/375°F/ gas mark 5.

Bring a small saucepan of water to the boil. Add a sprinkling of salt, 1 or 2 pierced garlic cloves and 1 whole lemon and boil for 5–10 minutes.

Remove the lemon from the pan and pierce it 10–15 times (you will need to wear gloves or hold the lemon still with a fork while you do this as the lemon will be hot). Stuff the lemon inside the chicken, along with the boiled garlic cloves, another 3 or 4 pierced garlic cloves, half the thyme and half the rosemary.

Put the chicken into a roasting tray with the carrots and parsnips around it. Lay the remaining rosemary, thyme and garlic cloves on top, then sprinkle with salt and pepper. Roast for 45 minutes.

Remove the tray from the oven, lift out the chicken and set aside. Toss the vegetables in the juices and herbs. Return the chicken to the tray, add the chicken stock and baste with some extra lemon juice. Return to the oven for a further 45 minutes until the chicken is cooked and its juices run clear.

Remove the chicken from the oven, discard the stuffing and carve.

Serve one portion of the chicken and vegetables with a Rainbow Salad. Keep one portion of the chicken for lunch the next day (*see* Chicken Salad on page 157) and either freeze the leftovers or use them in a Chunky Chicken Soup (*see* page 166).

Butter Bean & Courgetti Salad

Salads don't have to be boring. The butter beans have a delicate taste and let the other flavours do the talking, all while providing a healthy dose of dietary fibre, phytonutrients, protein and iron.

<u>2 servings</u>

300g (10½oz) tinned butter beans, drained and rinsed
200g (7oz) courgettes
1 head of Cos lettuce, shredded
2 shallots, finely diced
50g (1¾oz) fresh basil
juice of 2 lemons
50g (1¾oz) pine nuts
4 tablespoons extra virgin olive oil
3 tablespoons sunflower seeds
sea salt and cracked black pepper

Place the butter beans in a saucepan of hot water and bring to the boil. Reduce the heat and simmer for 2–3 minutes, then drain and allow to cool.

Using a spiralizer, prepare the courgetti. If you don't have a spiralizer, you can use a peeler to peel long, thin slices of courgette similar to tagliatelle.

Bring a saucepan of water to the boil. Drop in the courgetti and simmer for 1–2 minutes, then drain and allow to cool.

Place the lettuce, shallots, butter beans and courgetti in a large salad bowl.

In a blender, blitz the basil leaves, lemon juice, pine nuts and oil to a smooth, creamy consistency.

Drizzle the dressing over the salad, sprinkle with the sunflower seeds and season to taste with salt and pepper.

Divide into two portions. Serve one portion for dinner, and pack the other portion away in the fridge for lunch the next day.

Steak Strip Stir-fry

This simple stir-fry is packed full of flavour and is quick and easy to whip up.
The addition of detoxifying leafy greens and protein-rich quinoa means that it packs
a real punch, and is the perfect meal after a tough workout.

2 servings

90g (3^1/$_4$oz) quinoa (optional)
230ml (8fl oz) organic vegetable stock
3 tablespoons extra virgin olive oil
1 garlic clove, crushed
1 red onion, cut into wedges
250g (9oz) steak (grass-fed if available), sliced
1 teaspoon aluminium and gluten-free
   baking powder
1 red pepper, seeded and thinly sliced
2 courgettes, thinly sliced
2 large carrots, grated
100g (3^1/$_2$oz) kale, roughly chopped
150g (5^1/$_2$oz) spinach, chopped
80g (2^3/$_4$oz) tenderstem broccoli, chopped
1 teaspoon chilli powder
1 teaspoon dried oregano
1 teaspoon paprika
1 teaspoon ground cumin
2 tablespoons sunflower seeds
a squeeze of lemon juice (optional)
salt and cracked black pepper

If using the quinoa, put it into a saucepan with 230ml (8fl oz) of water and the vegetable stock. Bring to the boil, stir, then turn down to a simmer and cook for 5–7 minutes, or until light and fluffy. Wash well, then drain and set aside.

Meanwhile, heat 2 tablespoons of oil in a large wok. Add the garlic and onion, and lightly fry until golden brown.

Add the steak strips and sprinkle the baking powder over the slices, turning them over well with a wooden spoon or spatula. Once the strips are sealed on the outside, add the vegetables and the remaining tablespoon of oil and stir-fry, turning the contents of the wok over continuously. Add the salt, pepper, chilli powder, oregano, paprika and cumin as you continue to lightly stir-fry.

Once the vegetables have softened and the steak is cooked to your liking, add the cooked quinoa to the wok and gently heat through. Remove from the heat, tip half on to a plate and place the other half in a container for lunch the next day.

Sprinkle each serving with the sunflower seeds and a squeeze of lemon juice, if desired.

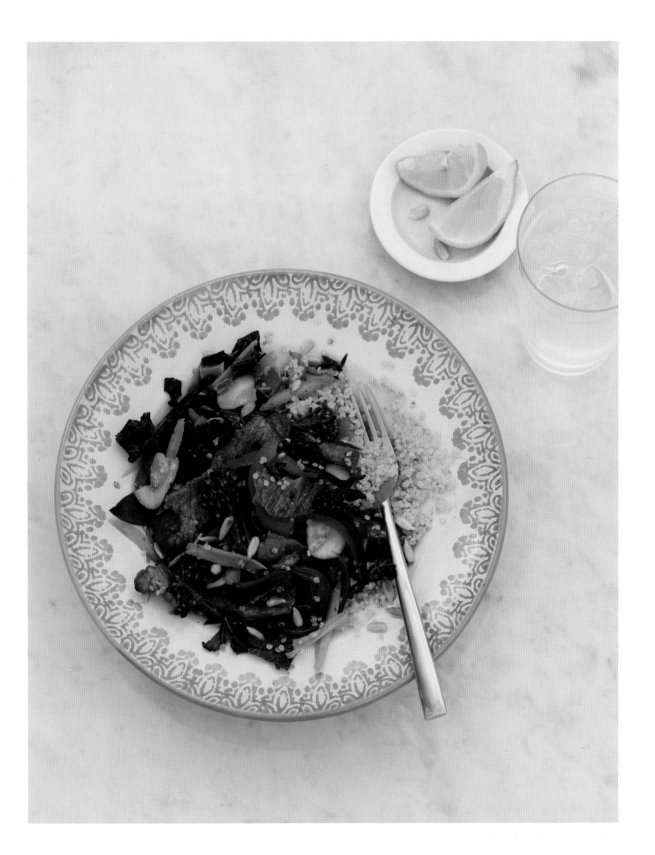

Turkey Burgers & Tandoori-roasted Cauliflower

Turkey is a source of lean protein and tastes delicious in these burgers, with spinach adding a hefty dose of iron, as well as vitamins A, C, E and K. The cauliflower is rich in anti-inflammatory spices and is perfect for anyone who likes a little spice.

2 servings

For the burgers

1 red onion, chopped

2 small garlic cloves, finely chopped

1 teaspoon dried rosemary

1 teaspoon turmeric

1 teaspoon paprika

3 fresh basil leaves, chopped

2 small handfuls of baby spinach

a small handful of watercress

zest of 1 lemon

1 teaspoon chia seeds

a pinch of coarse sea salt

1/2 teaspoon freshly ground black pepper

500g (1lb 2oz) turkey mince (I use thigh)

2 tablespoons extra virgin olive oil

Mixed Herb Salad, to serve (see page 191)

For the cauliflower steaks

1 large head of cauliflower, cut into slices lengthways

120g (4 1/4 oz) coconut yogurt

2 garlic cloves, crushed

1/2 teaspoon ground ginger

1/2 teaspoon ground cumin

1/2 teaspoon ground coriander

1/2 teaspoon paprika

1/2 teaspoon turmeric

1/2 teaspoon cayenne pepper (omit for a milder taste)

1/2 teaspoon salt

a pinch of cracked black pepper

juice of 1/2 lemon

Put the cauliflower steak ingredients into a large bowl and, using your hands, combine until the cauliflower is well coated. Cover the bowl, then marinate in the fridge for at least 1 hour, ideally overnight.

In a food processor, pulse together the burger ingredients, except the turkey mince and oil, then place the mixture in a large mixing bowl with the turkey and thoroughly combine. Form the mixture into 4 equal-sized patties and refrigerate for 1 hour.

Preheat the oven to 200°C/400°F/ gas mark 6. Line a baking tray with baking paper.

Put the cauliflower on the prepared tray and bake for 25–35 minutes, or until golden and slightly tender.

Heat a non–stick frying pan on a medium heat for about 1 minute, then add 1 teaspoon of oil and heat slightly. Add the burgers and cook for about 8–10 minutes on each side until browned and cooked through.

Serve 2 of the burgers with half the cauliflower steaks and a Mixed Herb Salad. Pack the other portion away for lunch the next day.

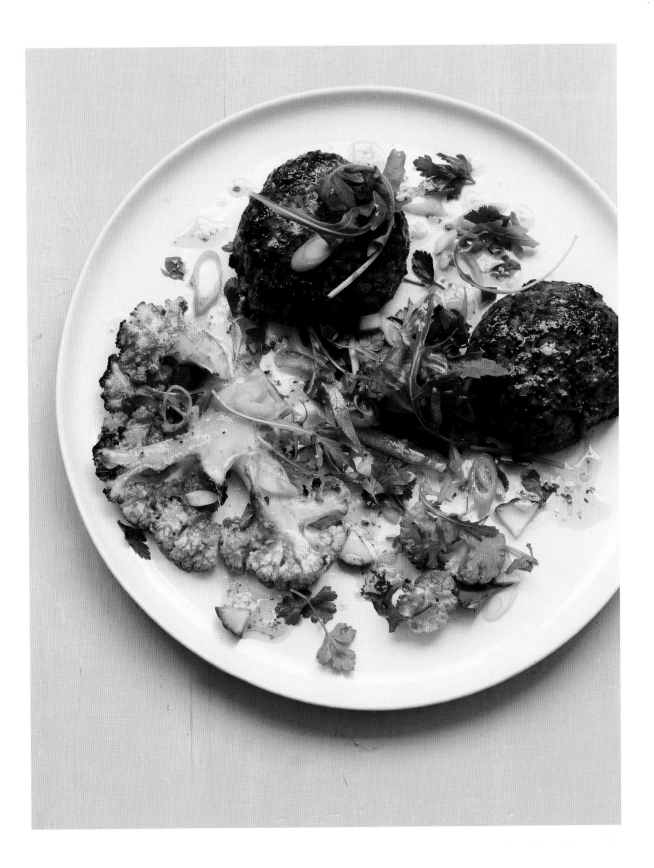

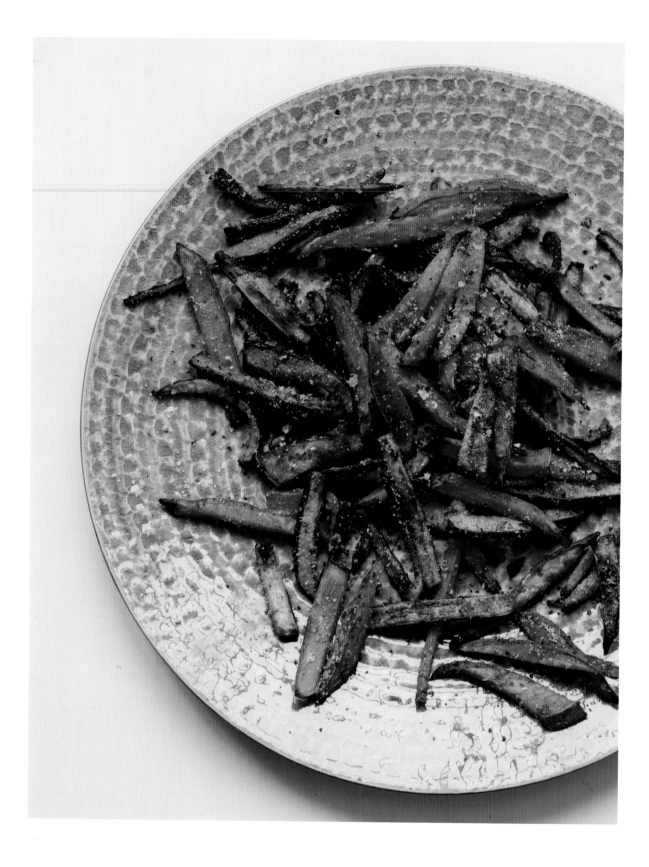

Baked Sweet Potato & Courgette Fries

These are a great side dish, and much healthier than frozen chips. Sweet potatoes are one of my favourite health carbs and are packed with vitamins and minerals, as well as body-loving fibre.

2 servings

1 medium sweet potato
1 large courgette
2 tablespoons extra virgin olive oil
2 teaspoons paprika
1 teaspoon garlic granules or crushed garlic
1 teaspoon coarse salt
cracked black pepper
a sprinkling of ground almonds

Preheat the oven to 220°C/425°F/ gas mark 7. Line a baking tray with baking paper.

Cut the potato and courgette into thin strips (I slice mine so that they are about 5mm/$^1/_4$ inch thick), or to your desired thickness.

Stir together the oil, paprika, garlic, salt and pepper in a large bowl. Toss the potato and courgette strips in the bowl, ensuring they are all evenly coated.

Drizzle a small amount of oil on to the prepared tray, then spread the vegetable strips on top in a single layer to ensure even cooking.

Bake for 25–30 minutes, turning the fries over twice during that time so that they cook evenly on all sides.

Add a sprinkling of ground almonds about 5 minutes before the fries are ready. When they start to crisp, remove the tray from the oven.

Serve with a sprinkling of coarse salt.

Crispy Roasted Chickpeas

Rich in phytonutrients, roasted chickpeas are a great alternative to an afternoon snack. Experiment with different herbs and spices to really make them your own.

4–6 servings

1 x 400g (14oz) BPA-free tin organic chickpeas, drained and rinsed

1 tablespoon extra virgin olive oil or melted coconut oil

1/2 teaspoon sea salt

1/2 tablespoon paprika

1/2 tablespoon ground cumin

Preheat the oven to 200°C/400°F/gas mark 6. Line a large baking tray with baking paper.

Pat the chickpeas completely dry – be patient and remove all the moisture, otherwise they won't crisp up.

Tip the chickpeas into a large bowl and toss with the oil and sea salt, ensuring they're evenly coated.

Tip the chickpeas on to the prepared tray and bake for about 25 minutes, stirring every 5 minutes or so until they are golden and crisp.

Remove the chickpeas from the oven and toss with the spices. Leave to cool, then store in an airtight container ready for snacking. The chickpeas will keep for up to 1 week.

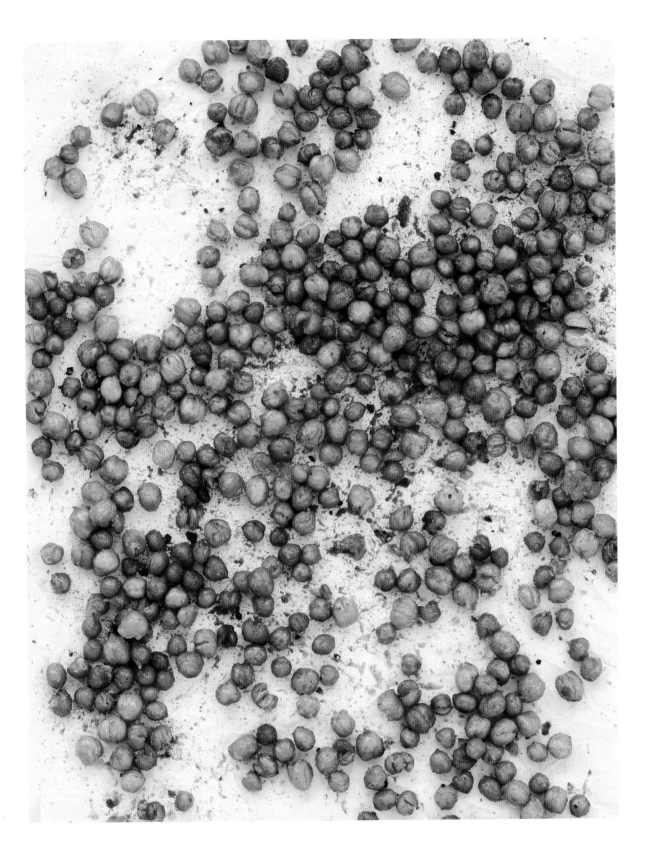

Hummus

If you're stuck for afternoon snack ideas, try making this delicious classic hummus and serving it with your favourite vegetables.

4 servings

1 x 400g (14oz) BPA-free tin of organic chickpeas, drained and rinsed

2 tablespoons extra virgin olive oil, plus extra to garnish

5–6 tablespoons raw tahini

1 garlic clove

1 teaspoon ground cumin

juice of 1 lemon

sea salt

Place all the ingredients in a blender or food processor and whiz to a paste.

If you are using a blender you may need to add small amounts of water as you go if the mixture is hard to blend – start by adding 100ml (3 1/2 fl oz) of cold water and gradually increase, 1 tablespoon at a time, if you find you need more. Be careful not to add too much, though, or your hummus will become watery.

Transfer to a small bowl and garnish with a drizzle of oil.

Serve chilled, with an assortment of your favourite freshly cut vegetables.

Red Pepper Hummus

This tasty spin on my classic hummus is sure to become one of your favourites. Red pepper adds a hefty dose of antioxidant vitamin C.

4 servings

1 large red pepper, halved lengthways, deseeded

1 x 400g (14oz) BPA-free tin of organic chickpeas, drained and rinsed

3–4 tablespoons extra virgin olive oil, plus extra to garnish

5–6 tablespoons raw tahini

1 garlic clove

juice of 1/2 lemon

1/2 teaspoon paprika, plus extra to garnish

sea salt

Preheat the grill to medium–high.

Place the pepper halves on a baking tray, cut-side down. Grill for about 15 minutes until the skins are blackened.

Transfer the peppers to a glass bowl, cover with a plate and leave to cool for 15–20 minutes. The steam will help to loosen their skins.

Once the peppers are cool enough to handle, peel off their skins. Don't worry if some blackened bits remain as this will add flavour.

Place the peppers in a blender or food processor with all the other ingredients and whiz to a paste. You may need to add a little water if the mixture is hard to blend – be careful not to add too much or your hummus will become watery.

Transfer to a small bowl and garnish with a drizzle of oil and a sprinkling of paprika.

Serve chilled, with an assortment of your favourite freshly cut vegetables.

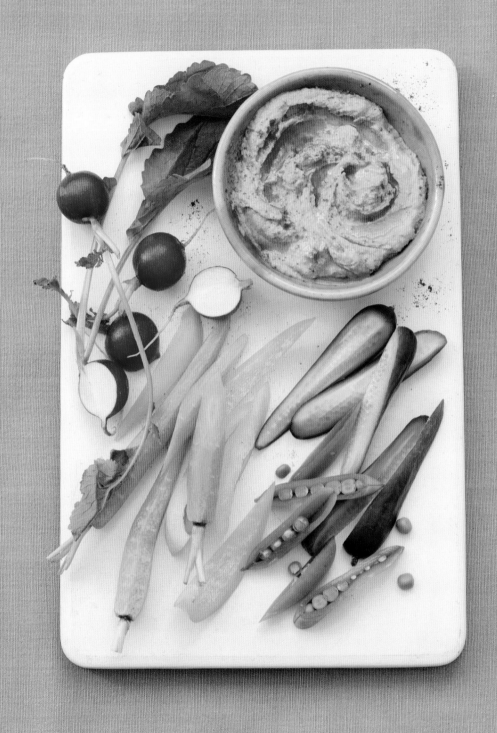

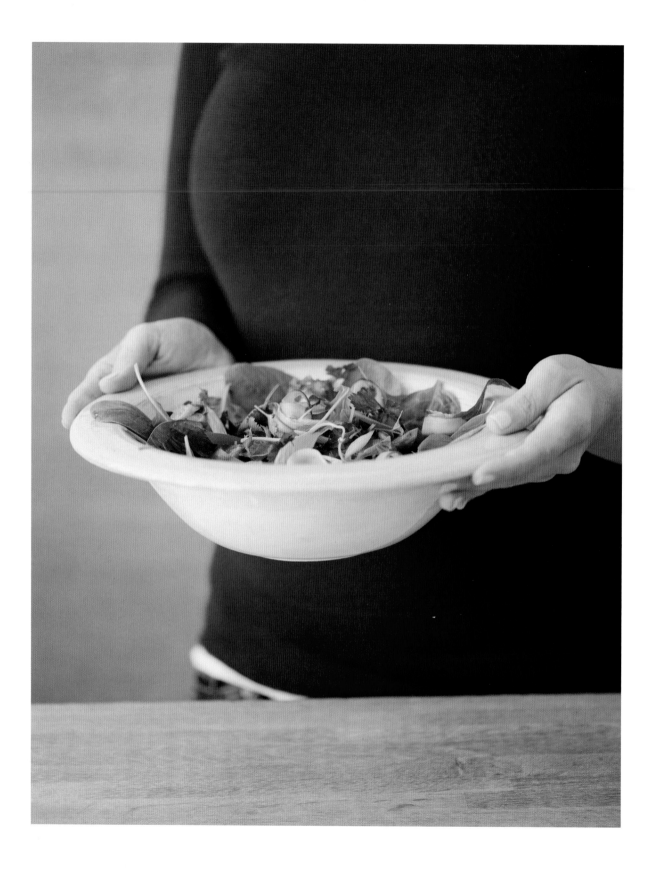

Mixed Herb Salad

Whether you want to serve it up as a side, toss it with some grilled meat or devour it on its own, this herby salad is full of flavour, fibre and antioxidants.

2 servings

For the salad

a handful of baby spinach

a handful of rocket

a small handful of fresh basil

a small handful of fresh coriander

a small handful of fresh flat-leaf parsley

a small bunch of spring onions, chopped

1 red pepper, thinly sliced

1/2 small cucumber, peeled into ribbons or chopped

For the dressing

3 1/2 tablespoons olive oil

2 tablespoons red wine vinegar

1 tablespoon Dijon mustard

1 tablespoon lemon juice

1 garlic clove, minced

1/2 teaspoon dried oregano

salt and pepper

Put all the salad ingredients into a large salad bowl.

Prepare the dressing by putting all the ingredients into a glass bowl or jar and stirring well. I like to use a glass jar with a lid and shake to combine everything.

Drizzle the dressing over the salad, then toss and enjoy. Store any leftover dressing in a jar in the fridge.

Chop Chop Salad (pictured)

Whenever you're in a hurry, grab these vibrant ingredients by the handful, toss them together and serve – a speedy, tasty salad that ticks all the boxes.

<u>1 serving</u>

2 handfuls of mixed salad leaves, chopped
1/4 cucumber, chopped
1 red pepper, deseeded and chopped
1 large vine tomato, chopped
1/2 ripe medium avocado, peeled and chopped
a small handful of fresh coriander, chopped
a small handful of fresh flat-leaf parsley, chopped
1/2 x 400g (14oz) BPA-free tin of chickpeas, drained and rinsed
1 teaspoon extra virgin olive oil
fresh lemon juice, to taste
a pinch of sea salt and cracked black pepper

Put all the ingredients into a large salad bowl and mix well.

Serve straight away, or as a side dish with your favourite meal.

Rainbow Salad

This salad is an easy way to add a rainbow to your diet – either eat it on its own or serve it alongside your favourite foods.

<u>2 servings</u>

1 head of Cos lettuce, chopped
1/2 cucumber, sliced
10 cherry tomatoes, halved
1/2 red onion, thinly sliced
1 green pepper, thinly sliced
juice of 1 lemon
1 tablespoon extra virgin olive oil
a pinch of salt and cracked black pepper

Put all the ingredients into a large salad bowl, then toss and serve. What could be easier?

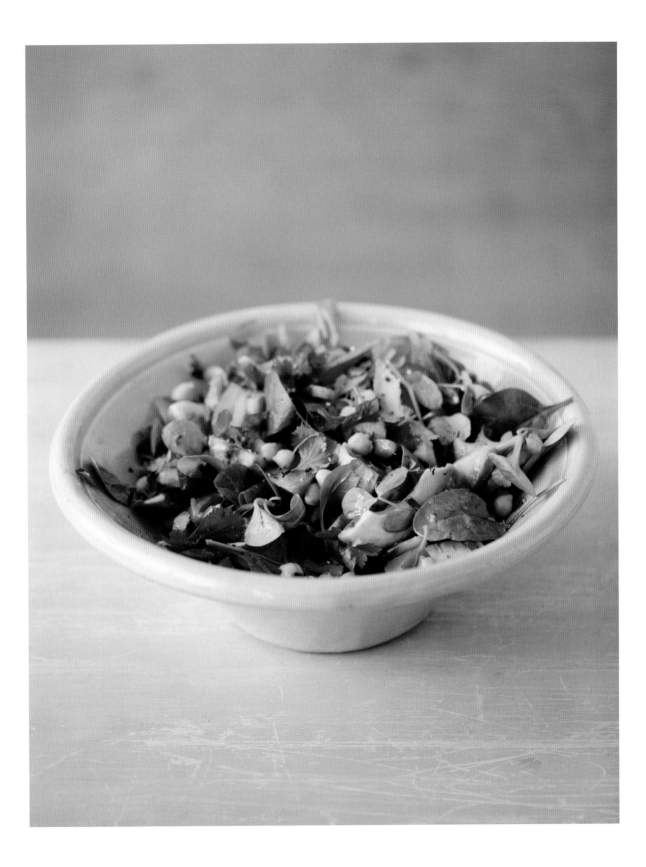

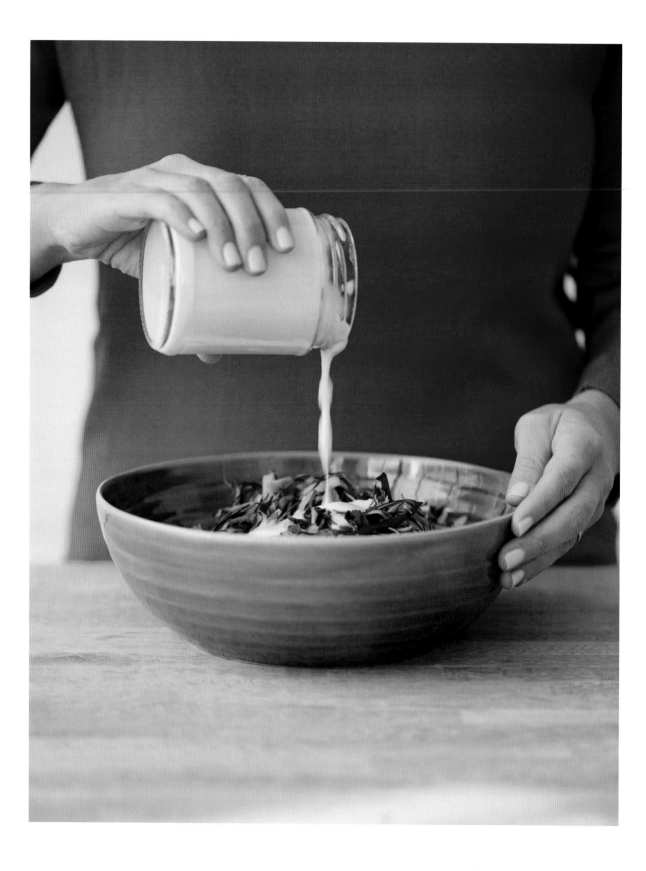

Purple Coleslaw

I've always loved coleslaw. My version uses fresh lime and herbs to pack a powerful phytonutrient punch, making it a great recipe for brightening up any lunchbox or salad.

4–6 servings

1 head of purple cabbage, shredded

2 large carrots, grated

1/2 bunch of fresh coriander, chopped

1/4 bunch of fresh flat-leaf parsley, chopped

200g (7oz) mayonnaise (vegan, homemade or plain)

7 tablespoons lime juice

1 1/2 tablespoons raw organic honey (optional)

sea salt and black pepper

Put all the vegetables and herbs into a large salad bowl and mix together.

In a separate bowl, combine the mayonnaise, lime juice and honey (if using). Season with salt and pepper, then pour the dressing over the vegetables and toss well.

Alternatively, you can prepare the dressing in advance and store it in a glass jar, ready to be used as needed.

Store the cabbage coleslaw in an airtight container in the fridge. Keeps for up to 5 days.

Sesame & Chilli Broccoli (pictured)

Leafy green broccoli is one of my most trusted detox warriors in hormone-balancing foods. Not only is this dish full of exotic flavours, but it will also help your body to regulate oestrogen, keeping everything in harmony.

2 servings

250g (9oz) tenderstem broccoli
1 tablespoon sesame seeds
1 fresh red chilli, finely chopped
1 tablespoon sesame oil
sea salt and cracked black pepper

Steam the broccoli for about 15 minutes. You can steam it for a longer or shorter time if you prefer, depending on how firm you like it. Drain if necessary, then allow it to steam-dry in a colander for 2–3 minutes.

Place the broccoli in a bowl and toss with the sesame seeds, chilli and sesame oil. Season with salt and pepper.

Steamed Spring Greens

Spring greens are a delicious light way of adding nutrient and fibre-packed veggies to your diet. A sprinkling of seeds adds crunch and a healthy dose of fats, too.

2 servings

400g (14oz) spring greens
1 tablespoon sesame seeds
1 tablespoon sunflower seeds
1 tablespoon pumpkin seeds
2 tablespoons extra virgin olive oil
juice of 1 lemon
sea salt and cracked black pepper

Cut the spring greens into strips about 5cm (2 inches) wide, being sure to remove the tough stems.

Steam the greens for about 5 minutes. Drain in a colander and set aside to allow to steam-dry before transferring to a serving bowl.

Add the seeds to the greens as they are or toast them in a pan for a couple of minutes first, turning them regularly to be sure not to burn them.

Put the oil, lemon juice, salt and black pepper into a glass jar and shake until well combined.

Pour the dressing over the greens, toss everything together and enjoy.

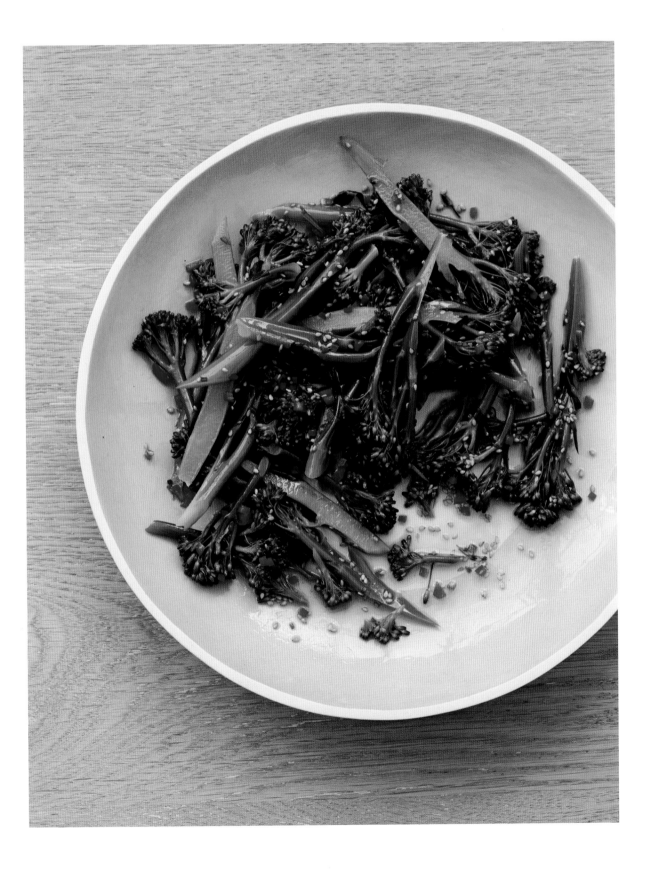

Steamed Greens

Body-loving broccoli is full of fibre, vitamins, calcium and iron. Rich in glucosinolates, it also helps liver detoxification, which in turn balances hormones by helping to clear toxins more effectively.

<u>2 servings</u>

200g (7oz) tenderstem broccoli
200g (7oz) green beans, trimmed
1 tablespoon extra virgin olive oil
2 garlic cloves, crushed
2 tablespoons tamari
1 tablespoon sesame seeds

Steam the greens for about 5 minutes until tender.

Meanwhile, heat the oil in a frying pan, then add the garlic and sauté until golden.

Toss the cooked greens with the garlic, then drizzle over the tamari and sauté for a further few minutes.

Sprinkle over the sesame seeds and serve immediately.

Steamed Chilli Greens

To keep bodies in balance, I recommend enjoying plenty of leafy, vibrant greens. Kale has become a real superhero in the food world, and it's perfect for helping our bodies to flush out any potential toxins and spent hormones.

<u>2 servings</u>

200g (7oz) tenderstem broccoli
200g (7oz) green beans, trimmed
150g (5^1/$_2$oz) kale
1 tablespoon extra virgin olive oil
2 garlic cloves, crushed
1 fresh red chilli, finely chopped
2 tablespoons tamari
a pinch of chilli flakes
1 tablespoon sesame seeds

Steam the greens for 5–8 minutes until tender.

Meanwhile, heat the oil in a frying pan, add the garlic and fresh chilli, and sauté until the garlic is golden.

Toss the cooked greens with the garlic and chilli, then drizzle over the tamari and sauté for a further few minutes.

Sprinkle over the chilli flakes and sesame seeds. Serve immediately.

Pistachio Pesto

One of my favourite herbs is antioxidant-rich basil, which is probably why I love pesto. This pistachio one is high in potassium and vitamin K.

4–6 servings

100g (3¹/₂oz) shelled pistachios
3 large handfuls of fresh basil
a handful of spinach
2 garlic cloves, finely chopped
juice of ¹/₂ lemon
100ml (3¹/₂fl oz) extra virgin olive oil
2 tablespoons nutritional yeast (optional)
sea salt and cracked black pepper

Place the pistachios in a blender and blitz until they are broken down and almost form a flour (or leave them chunkier, if you prefer).

Add the remaining ingredients and continue to blend until smooth, scraping down the sides and adding splashes of extra oil if needed, until you reach your desired consistency. Season to taste.

Store in a sealed glass jar in the fridge for up to 1 week. This pesto can also be frozen for up to 2 months for use another time.

Spinach & Cashew Pesto

The spinach in this pesto adds a hefty dose of phytonutrients and additional fibre, and is far tastier than store-bought varietes.

4–6 servings

a bunch of fresh basil leaves
zest and juice of 1 lemon
120ml (3³/₄fl oz) extra virgin olive oil
1 garlic clove, crushed
120g (4¹/₄oz) soaked cashew nuts, drained and patted dry
150g (5¹/₂oz) baby spinach, washed and roughly chopped
sea salt and black pepper

Blend all the ingredients together, keeping the mixture slightly chunky, adding salt and pepper to taste. Check the flavour and adjust as needed.

Store in a sealed glass jar in the fridge for up to 1 week, or divide between freezer bags and freeze for up to 2 months.

Simple Sauerkraut

Sauerkraut, a form of fermented cabbage, takes one of the world's healthiest probiotic foods and transforms it into something even healthier. You will also get vitamins C and K, calcium and potassium from this wonderful, gut-healing food.

**Makes a
1 litre jar**

1 head of green cabbage, sliced into
   thin ribbons
1½ tablespoons salt

Tip the cabbage into a large mixing bowl and sprinkle over the salt. Using your hands, massage the salt into the cabbage for 5–10 minutes until the cabbage becomes slightly limp.

Take handfuls of the cabbage and press them tightly into a sterilized 1-litre mason jar. Pour over any liquid you created when massaging the cabbage, then screw on the lid.

Over the course of the next day, remove the lid and press down on the cabbage at least four times. The cabbage should become more limp, and its liquid will eventually rise above it. If, after 24 hours, there's not enough liquid to cover the cabbage, dissolve 1 teaspoon of salt in 200ml (7fl oz) of water and pour in enough to cover.

Ferment in a cool, dark place for at least 3 days. Taste the cabbage and, if it tastes good to you, pop it into the fridge and eat it alongside meals. If you want to ferment it for longer, put it back in a cool, dark place.

Sauerkraut will keep for several months in the fridge.

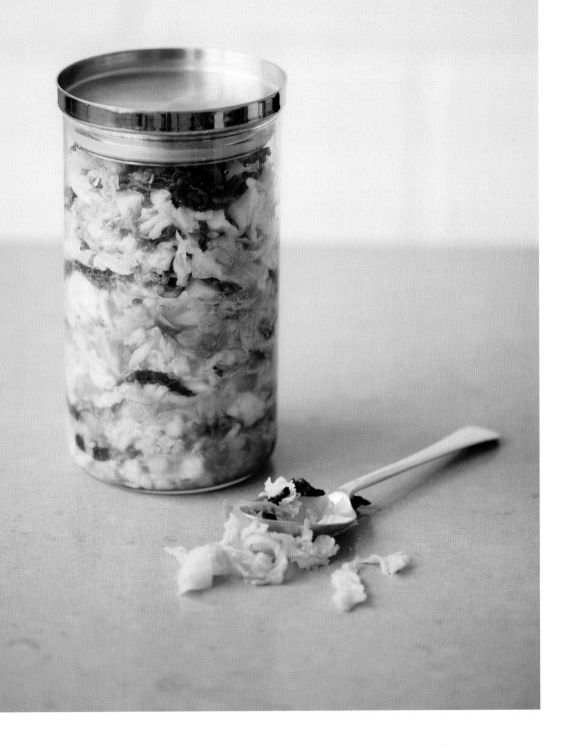

Almond & Cashew Protein Balls

These delicious protein balls are packed with fibre and healthy fats to keep you full and satisfied, and are ideal for stashing in your handbag for a healthy snack.

Makes 12–15

50g (1³/₄oz) raw almonds

100g (3¹/₂oz) raw cashews

3 tablespoons coconut oil, melted

30g (1oz) almond flour

30g (1oz) unsweetened desiccated coconut, plus extra for rolling (optional)

³/₄ teaspoon ground cinnamon

1 teaspoon pure vanilla extract or vanilla powder

90g (3¹/₄oz) dried unsweetened apricots, chopped

Place the almonds and cashews in a large bowl. Cover them with hot water and leave to soak for 30 minutes, then drain and pat dry.

Put the soaked nuts into a blender or processor and process to a thick paste, scraping down the sides of the blender as you go.

Add the melted coconut oil to the blender and process until the mixture has a nut-butter-like texture.

Add the remaining ingredients, apart from the apricots, and process gently to combine. Then add the apricots and process just enough to mix them in.

Take 1 tablespoon of mixture for each ball, rolling it in your hands to make 12–15 balls. I find wetting my hands makes the balls easier to roll.

You can roll the balls in extra desiccated coconut, if you like.

Store in an airtight container in the fridge for up to 1 week, or in the freezer for up to 3 months.

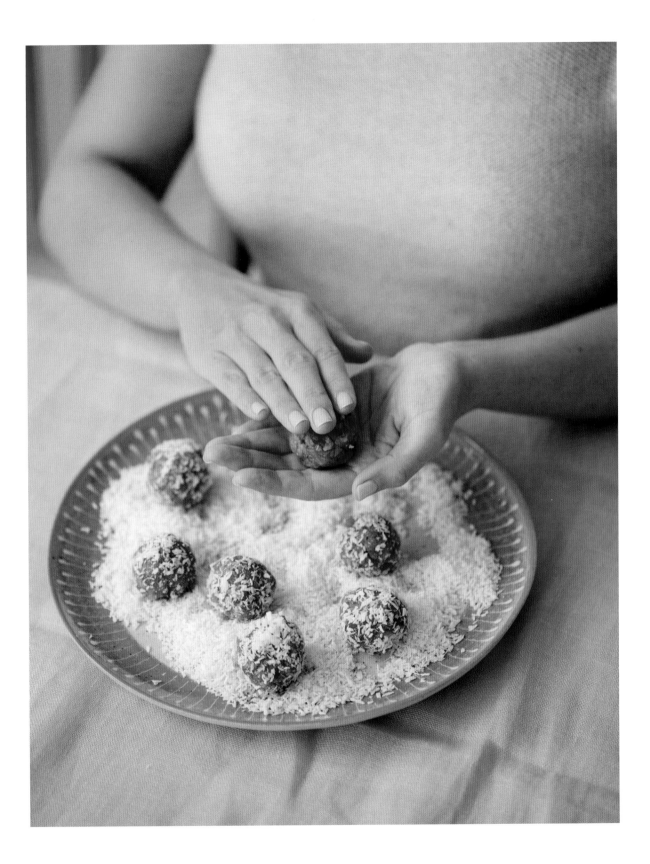

Baked Apples with Vanilla Cashew Cream

There's something so comforting about a sweet, baked apple, and it tastes extra special when served with spoonfuls of my vanilla cashew cream. Full of vitamins, minerals and healthy fats, and a great way to use up any older apples.

2 servings

2 large apples of choice
1 1/2 teaspoons raw honey
a drizzle of lemon juice
1/2 teaspoon coconut oil, melted
1/4 teaspoon ground cinnamon
4 tablespoons chopped walnuts, to serve

For the vanilla cashew cream

140g (5oz) cashews, soaked in water for 3–4 hours, then drained
1 date (optional)
3 1/2 tablespoons coconut milk (or water)
juice of 1/4 lemon
seeds from 1 vanilla pod, or 1 tablespoon sugar-free vanilla extract
a pinch of sea salt

Preheat the oven to 180°C/350°F/ gas mark 4. Line a baking tray with greaseproof paper.

Using a sharp knife, carefully slice the top off each apple. Place them on the prepared tray and drizzle over the honey, lemon juice and coconut oil, then sprinkle with the cinnamon. Bake for 20–30 minutes, or until softened and the juices are oozing.

Meanwhile, make the cashew cream by putting all the ingredients into a blender and blitzing until smooth, scraping down the sides of the blender as you go. Add a splash more water or coconut milk, if needed, until you reach the desired consistency.

Once ready to serve, spoon the cashew cream over the apples and sprinkle with the chopped walnuts.

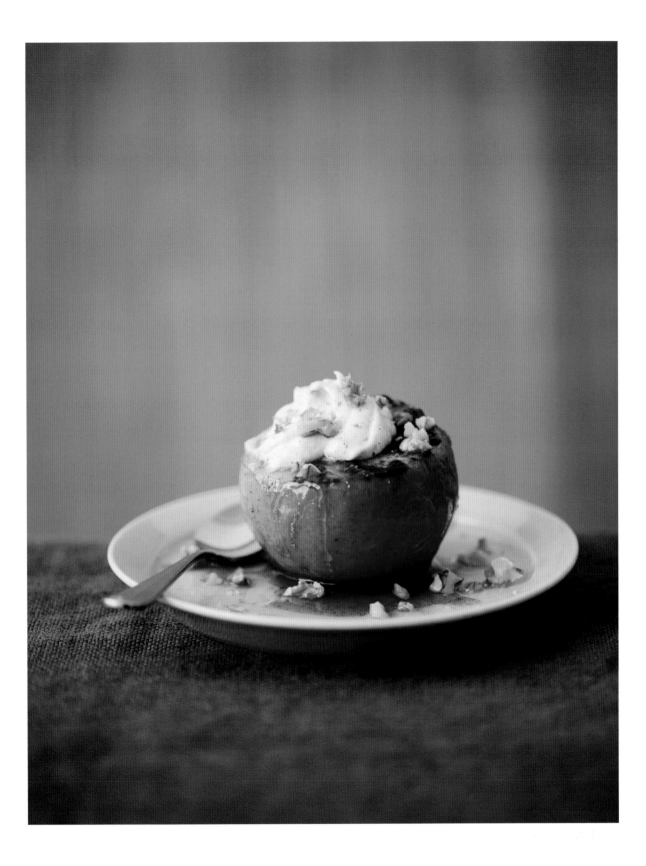

Banana Nice Creams

Many of my clients have commented that nothing tastes better than a sweet, chocolatey ice cream. With that in mind, I created these healthy ices that taste great and help to supply your body with hormone-balancing healthy fats.

6 servings

For the ice cream

1 x 400ml (14fl oz) BPA-free tin of full-fat coconut milk, chilled in the fridge overnight

3 bananas, chopped and frozen

1½ teaspoons vanilla paste or sugar-free vanilla extract

For the chocolate coating

200g (7oz) dark chocolate or cacao nibs (75% cacao solids or above), finely chopped

2 teaspoons coconut oil

Start by making the ice cream. Blend all the ingredients together until smooth, then spoon into silicone ice cream moulds. Insert the sticks and place in the freezer to set overnight, or for about 6 hours.

Once your ice creams have set, make the chocolate coating. Melt together the dark chocolate and coconut oil in a bain-marie. Stir frequently until melted and smooth, then take off the heat and set aside to cool slightly.

Remove the ice creams from the freezer and dunk each one into the melted chocolate, turning to coat. Hold each ice cream until the coating has set (it shouldn't take long), then lay them on a baking tray.

Eat immediately, or return them to the freezer until ready to enjoy.

Chocolate Coconut Cream

This is so addictive that you'll soon be eating it straight from the freezer. Happily, the sweetness comes from fibrous dates, and the cacao powder will give your body a delicious dose of antioxidants, as well as a happy endorphin boost.

<u>4–6 servings</u>

1 x 400ml (14fl oz) BPA-free tin of full-fat coconut milk, chilled in the fridge overnight

4$\frac{1}{2}$ tablespoons raw cacao powder

6 medjool dates, pitted, or 3 tablespoons pure maple syrup

$\frac{1}{2}$ teaspoon vanilla extract

a pinch of salt

100g (3$\frac{1}{2}$oz) cacao nibs (at least 75% cacao solids or above)

Toppings (optional)
grain-free granola

fresh berries

Line a loaf tin with foil.

Blend together all the ingredients, except the cacao nibs, in a blender until completely smooth and creamy.

Taste and adjust the sweetness by adding more dates or maple syrup, if necessary, then stir through the cacao nibs.

Pour into the prepared loaf tin (or ice cream moulds) and cover with foil. Leave to set for at least 4–6 hours, ideally overnight.

Remove from the freezer at least 15 minutes before serving, then enjoy.

Fruit Salad & Coconut Yogurt

*Full of natural sweetness from the fruit and with some added fats in the form
of coconut yogurt and seeds, this is one of my favourite desserts to make.*

<u>1 serving</u>

5 heaped tablespoons coconut yogurt
5 raspberries
2 strawberries, sliced
5–10 blueberries
½ plum, sliced
½ small apple, diced
1 teaspoon sunflower seeds
1 tablespoon ground flax seeds
1 teaspoon ground cinnamon

Put the yogurt into a bowl and top
with the fruit.

Sprinkle with the seeds and cinnamon,
and serve.

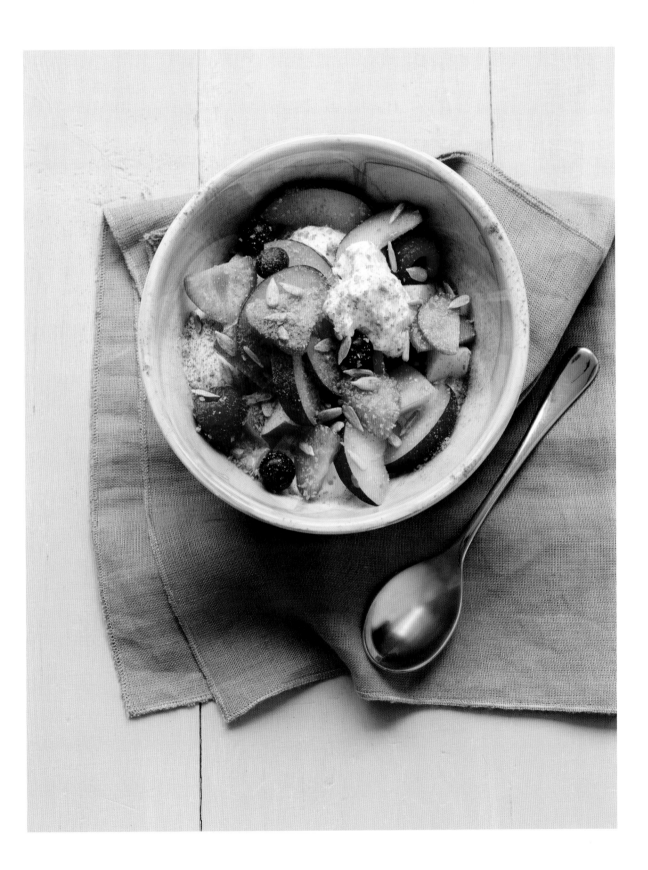

Tartes aux Citron

Fans of this light and airy French pudding will love the melt-in-the-mouth pastry and zesty filling. It might just be love at first bite.

4 servings

For the pastry

280g (10oz) almond flour

2 tablespoons arrowroot

2 tablespoons coconut oil, plus extra
   for greasing

1 tablespoon maple syrup or raw honey

1 egg

2 tablespoons maca powder (optional)

a pinch of salt

For the filling

3 eggs

3 tablespoons raw honey

6 tablespoons lemon juice (or more, to taste)

4 tablespoons coconut oil

zest of 1 lemon, plus extra to serve (optional)

1/2 teaspoon turmeric

a drop of lemon extract (optional)

2 tablespoons maca powder (optional)

a pinch of sea salt

Preheat the oven to 180°C/350°F/ gas mark 4. Grease 4 small tart cases.

Mix together all the pastry ingredients until they form a dough, then press into the base of your tins, being sure to line the sides, too. Prick the pastry all over with a fork, then bake for about 8 minutes, or until golden.

Make the filling by gently whisking together all the ingredients in a bowl. Pour into a saucepan and place on a low heat, whisking constantly for about 5 minutes until the mixture thickens (don't stop whisking, otherwise the eggs will scramble).

Taste and add more lemon if desired. Remove from the heat, then blend until smooth, if necessary.

Leave to cool, then spoon the filling into the tart cases. Place in the fridge to chill or eat straight away. Scatter with extra lemon zest before serving, if liked.

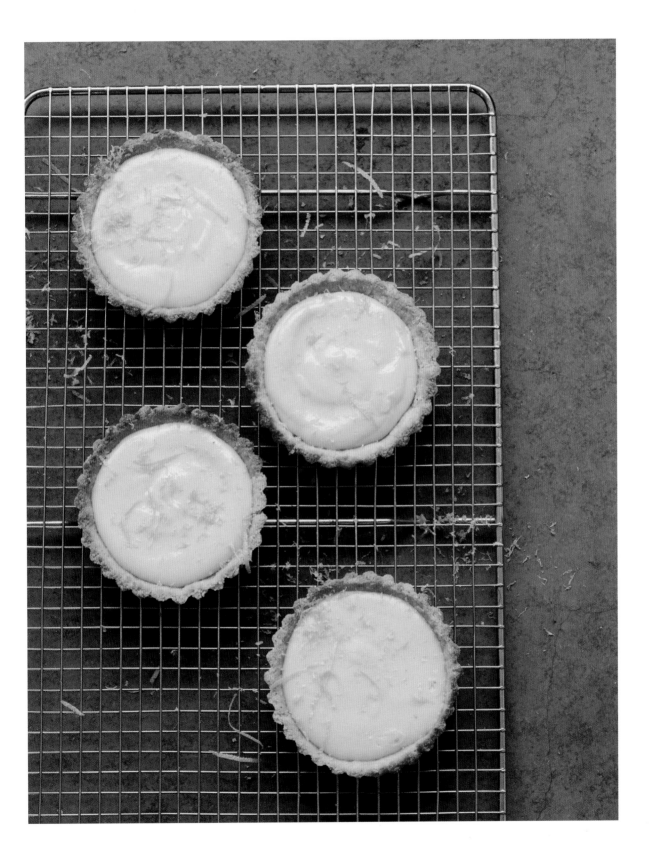

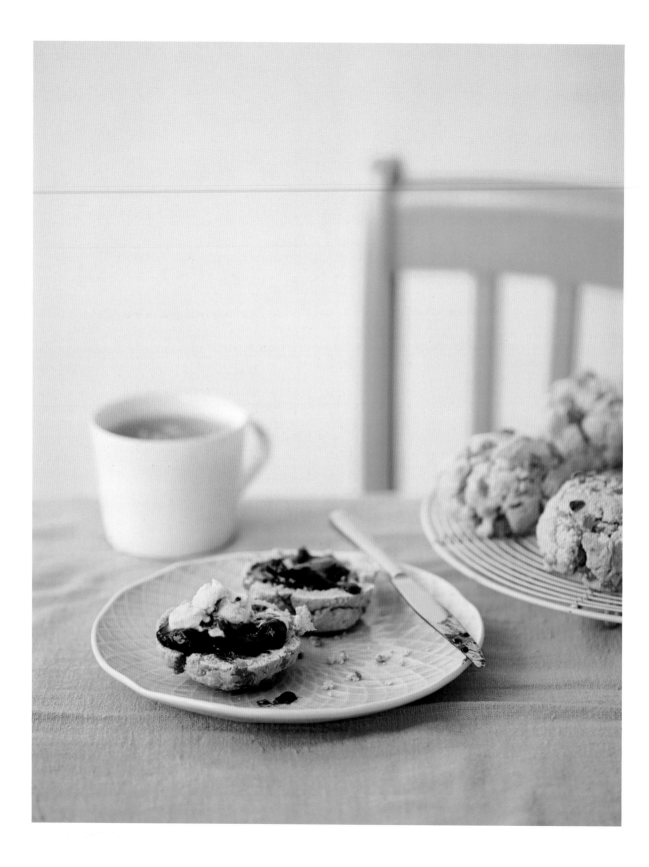

Scones with Cashew Cream & Chia Jam

These gluten-free scones are made with almond flour, which can help to balance hormone production, and fibre-rich coconut flour. I love serving them with lashings of cashew cream and some fruity chia jam for the perfect afternoon tea.

<u>8 servings</u>
(makes 4 scones)

175g (6oz) almond flour
3 tablespoons coconut flour
1 tablespoon arrowroot
1/2 teaspoon bicarbonate of soda
a pinch of salt
1 large organic free-range egg
3 tablespoons maple syrup or raw honey
1 1/2 teaspoons vanilla paste
1 tablespoon almond milk, plus 1 tablespoon to glaze
80g (2 3/4oz) unsweetened dried apricots, chopped (optional)

To serve
Chia Jam (*see* page 119)
Cashew Cream (*see* page 204)

Preheat the oven to 170°C/325°F/ gas mark 3. Line a baking tray with greaseproof paper.

Stir together all the dry ingredients in a large mixing bowl.

In a separate bowl, beat the egg with the maple syrup, vanilla and 1 tablespoon of almond milk until smooth.

Stir the wet ingredients into the dry ingredients until just combined, adding a splash more milk or water if the mixture feels too dry, then stir in the dried apricots if using.

Shape the dough into 4 scones. Brush over the additional tablespoon of almond milk and bake for 20–30 minutes, or until golden.

Allow the scones to cool slightly until easy to handle, or cool completely if serving cold.

Serve the scones with dollops of cream and jam and a good mug of herbal tea.

References

Part 1 – How Hormones Work

Hiller-Sturmhöfel S and Bartke A (1998) "The endocrine system: An overview", *Alcohol Health Research World*, vol. 22, pp.153–64

"Hypothyroidism: symptoms" (8 October 2014) *Pub Med Health: Glossary*

"Overactive thyroid: overview" (9 October 2014) *Pub Med Health: Glossary*

Davis S (2001) "Testosterone deficiency in women", *Journal of Reproductive Medicine*, vol. 46, pp.291–96

Riedel-Baima B and Riedel A (2008) "Female pattern hair loss may be triggered by low oestrogen to androgen ratio", *Endocrine Regulations*, vol.42, pp.14–16

Vallee M (2016) "Neurosteroids and potential therapeutics: Focus on pregnenolone", *Journal of Steroid Biochemistry and Molecular Biology*, vol. 160, pp.78–87

Wilcox G (2005) "Insulin and insulin resistance", *Clinical Biochemist Reviews*, vol. 26, pp.19–39

Progesterone

Kondoru L (2012) "Biomarkers of chronic stress", *Master's Thesis, University of Pittsburgh*

Seifert-Klauss V and Prior J C (2010) "Progesterone and bone: Actions promoting bone health in women", *Journal of Osteoporosis*, vol. 2010, pp.1–18

Testosterone

Panzer C et al (2006) "Impact of oral contraceptives on sex hormone-binding globulin and androgen levels: a retrospective study in women with sexual dysfunction", *Journal of Sexual Medicine*, vol. 3, pp.104–13

Zimmerman Y *et al* (2014) "The effect of combined oral contraception on testosterone levels in healthy women: a systematic review and meta-analysis" *Human Reproduction Update*, vol. 20, pp.76–105

Oestrogen

Bretveld R W *et al* (2006) "Pesticide exposure: the hormonal system of the female reproductive system disrupted?" *Reproductive Biology and Endocrinology*, vol. 4, pp.30

Lokuge S *et al* (2011) "Depression in women: windows of vulnerability and new insights into the link between estrogen and serotonin", *Journal of Clinical Psychiatry*, vol. 72, pp.1563–69

Rossignol A M (1985) "Caffeine-containing beverages and premenstrual syndrome in young women", *American Journal of Public Health*, vol. 75, pp.1335–37

Williams G P (2010) "The role of oestrogen in the pathogenesis of obesity, type 2 diabetes, breast cancer and prostate disease", *European Journal of Cancer*, vol. 19, pp.256–71

Usdan L S *et al* (2008) "The endocrinopathies of anorexia nervosa", *Endocrine Practice*, vol. 14, pp.1055–63

Cortisol

Barron M L (2007) "Light exposure, melatonin secretion, and menstrual cycle parameters: an integrative review", *Biological Research for Nursing*, vol. 9, pp.49–69

Kollipaka R *et al* (2013) "Does psychosocial stress influence menstrual abnormalities in medical students?", *Journal of Obstetrics and Gynaecology*, vol. 33, pp.489–93

Kyrou I *et al* (2006) "Stress, visceral obesity and metabolic complications", *Annals of the New York Academy of Sciences*, vol. 1083, pp.77–110

Torres S J and Nowson C A (2007) "Relationship between stress, eating behavior, and obesity", *Nutrition*, vol. 23, pp.887–94

Yamamoto K *et al* (2009) "The relationship between premenstrual symptoms, menstrual pain, irregular menstrual cycles, and psychosocial stress among Japanese college students", *Journal of Physiological Anthropology*, vol. 28, pp.129–36

Thyroid

Brent G A (2010) "Environmental exposures and autoimmune thyroid disease", Thyroid, vol. 20, pp.755–61

Tsigos C and Chrousos G P (2002) "Hypothalamic-pituitary-adrenal axis, neuroendocrine factors and stress", Journal of Psychosomatic Research, vol. 53, pp.865–71

Insulin

Ahmad J et al (2006) "Inflammation, insulin resistance and carotid IMT in first degree relatives of north Indian type 2 diabetic subjects", Diabetes Research in Clinical Practice, vol. 73, pp.205–10

Bergman B C et al (2012) "Novel and reversible mechanisms of smoking-induced insulin resistance in humans", Diabetes, vol. 61, pp.3156–66

Triplitt C L (2012) "Examining the mechanisms of glucose regulation", American Journal of Managed Care, vol. 18, pp.S4–10

Part 2 – Showstoppers

Bretveld R W *et al* (2006) "Pesticide exposure: the hormonal system of the female reproductive system disrupted?" *Reproductive Biology and Endocrinology*, vol. 4, pp.30

Gallo M V *et al* (2016) "Endocrine disrupting chemicals and ovulation: Is there a relationship?" *Environmental Research*, vol. 151, pp.410–18

Kuch H M and Ballschmiter K (2001) "Determination of endocrine-disrupting phenolic compounds and estrogens in surface and drinking water by HRGC-(NCI)-MS in the picogram per liter range", *Environmental Science and Technology*, vol. 35, pp.3201–06.

Lopez-Carrillo *et al* (2010) "Exposure to phthalates and breast cancer risk in Northern Mexico", *Environmental Health Perspectives*, vol. 118.4, pp.539–44

Lorber M *et al* (2015) "Exposure assessment of adult intake of bisphenol A (BPA) with emphasis on canned food dietary exposures", *Environment International*, vol. 77, pp.55–62

Michalowicz J (2014) " Bisphenol A: sources, toxicity and biotransformation", *Environmental Toxicity and Pharmacology*, vol. 37, pp.738–58

Roy J R *et al* (2009) "Estrogen-like endocrine disrupting chemicals affecting puberty in humans – a review", *Medical Science Monitor*, vol. 15, pp.137–45

Premenstrual Syndrome (PMS)

Greene R and Dalton K (1953) "The premenstrual syndrome", *British Medical Journal*, vol. 1 (4818)

Yonkers K A et al (2008) "Premenstrual syndrome", *The Lancet*, vol. 371, pp.1200–10

The Modern Diet

Liska D A J (1998) "The detoxification enzyme systems", *Alternative Medicine Review*, vol. 3, pp.187–98

Macintosh A and Ball K.(2000) "The effects of a short program of detoxification in disease free individuals", *Alternative Therapies in Health and Medicine*, vol. 6.4, pp.70–76

Chronic Stress

Grandi G *et al* (2016) "Inflammation influences steroid hormone receptors targeted by progestins in endometrial stromal cells from women with endometriosis", *Journal of Reproductive Immunology*, vol. 117, pp.30–38

Poor Elimination

Collins S M *et al* (2012) "The interplay between the intestinal microbiota and the brain", *Nature Reviews Microbiology*, vol. 10, pp.735–42

PCOS & Endometriosis

Bulun S E *et al* (2002) "Mechanisms of excessive estrogen formation in endometriosis", *Journal of Reproductive Immunology*, vol. 55, pp.21–33

"Endometriosis symptoms" (7 May 2014), *Pub Med Health*

Kitawaki J *et al* (2002) "Endometriosis: The pathophysiology as an estrogen dependent disease", *Journal of Steroid Biochemistry and Molecular Biology*, vol. 83, pp.149–55

Straub R H (2006) "The complex role of estrogens in inflammation", *Endocrine Reviews*, vol. 28, pp.521–74

Tremellen K, Pearce K (2012) "Dysbiosis of gut microbiota (DOGMA) – a novel theory for the development of polycystic ovarian syndrome", *Medical Hypotheses*, vol. 79, pp.104–12

Part 3 – The Six Pillars of Balance

Pillar One: Nourish/Eat Real Whole Food not Processed Junk Food

Miles I A (2014) "Fast food fever: Reviewing the impacts of the Western diet on immunity", *Nutrition Journal*, vol. 13:61.

Pillar One: Nourish/Eat the Right Carbs, Not No Carbs

Chavarro J E *et al* (2009) "A prospective study of dietary carbohydrate quantity and quality in relation to risk of ovulatory infertility", *European Journal of Clinical Nutrition*, vol. 63, pp.78–86

Collier B *et al* (2008) "Glucose control and the inflammatory response", *Nutrition in Clinical Practice*, vol. 23, pp.3–15

Gross L S *et al* (2004) "Increased consumption of refined carbohydrates and the epidemic of type 2 diabetes in the United States: an ecologic assessment", *American Journal of Clinical Nutrition*, vol. 79, pp.774–79

Johnson R K et al (2009) "Dietary sugars intake and cardiovascular health: a scientific statement from the American Heart Association", *Circulation*, vol. 120, pp.1011–20

Pillar One: Nourish/Eat a Rainbow of Vegetables

Aune D *et al* (2017) "Fruit and vegetable intake and the risk of cardiovascular disease, total cancer and all-cause mortality – a systematic review and dose-response meta-analysis of prospective studies", *International Journal of Epidemiology*.

Slavin J L and Lloyd B (2012) "Health benefits of fruits and vegetables", *Advances in Nutrition*, vol. 3, pp.503–16

Pillar One: Nourish/Have a Green Smoothie a Day

Long S and Romani A M P (2015) "Role of cellular magnesium in human diseases. *Austin Journal of Nutrition and Food Science*, vol. 2, pp.1051

Pillar One: Nourish/Stay Hydrated

Jequier E and Constant F (2010) "Water as an essential nutrient: the physiological basis of hydration", *European Journal of Clinical Nutrition*, vol. 64, pp.115–23

Pillar One: Nourish/Avoid Caffeine, Alcohol and Stimulants

Bergmann MM, *et al* (2011) "The association of lifetime alcohol use with measures of abdominal and general adiposity in a large-scale European cohort", *European Journal of Clinical Nutrition*, vol. 65, pp.1079–87

Emanuele N and Emanuele M A (1997) "The endocrine system: alcohol alters critical hormonal balance", *Alcohol Health Research World*, vol. 21, pp.53–64

Gold E B, *et al* (2007) "Diet and lifestyle factors associated with premenstrual symptoms in a racially diverse community sample: Study of Women's Health Across the Nation (SWAN)", *Journal of Women's Health*, vol. 16, pp.641–56

Rachdaoui N and Sarkar D K (2013) "Effects of alcohol on the endocrine system", *Endocrinology and Metabolism Clinics of North America*, vol. 42, pp.593–615

Rossignol A M.(1985) "Caffeine-containing beverages and premenstrual syndrome in young women", *American Journal of Public Health*, vol. 75, pp.1335–37

Sarkola T *et al* (1999) "Acute effect of alcohol on estradiol, estrone, progesterone, prolactin, cortisol, and luteinizing hormone in premenopausal women", *Alcoholism Clinical and Experimental Research*, vol. 23, pp.976–82

Suez J *et al* (2014) "Artificial sweeteners induce glucose intolerance by altering the gut microbiota", *Nature*, vol. 514, pp.181–86

Pillar One: Nourish/Go Organic as Much as Your Budget Allows

Leifert C *et al* (2014) "Higher antioxidant and lower cadmium concentrations and lower incidence of pesticide residues in organically grown crops: a systematic literature review and meta-analyses", *British Journal of Nutrition*, vol. 112, pp.794–811

Pillar One: Nourish/Say No to Gluten…

Antvorskov J C *et al* (2012) "Dietary gluten alters the balance of pro-inflammatory and anti-inflammatory cytokines in T cells of BALB/c mice", *Immunology*, vol. 138, pp.23–33

Herfarth H H *et al* (2014) "Prevalence of a gluten free diet and improvement of clinical symptoms in patients with inflammatory bowel diseases", *Inflammatory Bowel Disease*, vol. 20, pp.1194–97

Soares F L *et al* (2013) "Gluten-free diet reduces adiposity, inflammation and insulin resistance associated with the induction of PPAR-alpha and PPAR-gamma expression", *Journal of Nutritional Biochemistry*, vol. 24, pp.1105–11

Pillar One: Nourish/…and Dairy

Ganmaa D, Sato A (2005) "The possible role of female sex hormones in milk from pregnant cows in the development of breast, ovarian and corpus uteri cancers", *Medical Hypotheses*, vol. 65, pp.1028–37

Malekinejad M and Rezabakhsh A (2015) "Hormones in dairy foods and their impact on public health: A narrative review article", *Iran Journal of Public Health*, vol. 44, pp.742–58

Pillar Two: Balance/12 Steps to Jumping off the Blood-sugar Roller-coaster

Add Good-quality protein to Every Meal or Snack

Cannon M C *et al* (2003) "An increase in dietary protein improves the blood glucose response in persons with type 2 diabetes", *American Journal of Clinical Nutrition*, vol. 78, pp.734–41

Avoid Sugar or Synthetic Sweeteners

Anderson R A (2008) "Chromium and polyphenols from cinnamon improve insulin sensitivity", *Proceedings of the Nutrition Society*, vol. 67, pp.48–53

Mang B *et al* (2006) "Effects of a cinnamon extract on plasma glucose, HbA, and serum lipids in diabetes mellitus type 2", *European Journal of Clinical Investigation*, vol. 36, pp.340–44

Yang Q (2010) "Gain weight by 'going diet?' Artificial sweeteners and the neurobiology of sugar cravings", *Yale Journal of Biology and Medicine*, vol. 83, pp.101–08

Get Moving

Bourghouts L B and Keizer H A (2000) "Exercise and insulin sensitivity: A review", *International Journal of Sports Medicine*, vol. 21, pp.1–12

Avoid Stimulants

Lovallo W R *et al* (2006) "Cortisol responses to mental stress, exercise, and meals following caffeine intake in men and women", *Pharmacological Biochemistry and Behaviour*, vol. 83, pp.441–47

Pillar Two: Balance/Gut Health

Bae S H (2014) "Diets for constipation", *Paediatric, Gastroenterology, Hepatology & Nutrition*, vol. 17, pp.203–08

Gold E B *et al* (2016) "The association of inflammation with pre-menstrual symptoms", *Journal of Women's Health*, vol. 25, pp.865–74

Jungbauer A and Mediakovic S (2012) "Anti-inflammatory properties of culinary herbs and spices that ameliorate the effects of metabolic syndrome" *Maturitas*, vol. 71, pp.227–39

Kiecolt-Glaser J K (2010) "Stress, food, and inflammation: Psychoneuroimmunology and nutrition at the cutting edge", *Psychosomatic Medicine*, vol. 72, pp.365–69

West C E *et al* (2015) "The gut microbiota and inflammatory noncommunicable diseases: associations and potentials for gut microbiota therapies", *Journal of Allergy and Clinical Immunology*, vol. 135, pp.3–13

Pillar Two: Balance/Eight Principles for Better Digestion

Eco-warriors

Vermorken A J M et al (2016) "Bowel movement frequency, oxidative stress and disease prevention", *Molecular and Clinical*

Oncology, vol. 5, pp.339–42

Fibre

Anderson J W *et al* (2009) "Health benefits of dietary fiber", *Nutrition Reviews*, vol. 67, pp.188–205

Pillar Three: Nurture/Prioritise Sleep

AlDabal L and BaHammam A S (2011) "Metabolic, endocrine, and immune consequences of sleep deprivation", Open Respiratory Medicine Journal, vol. 5, pp.31–43

Jung C M *et al* (2010) "Acute effects of bright light exposure on cortisol levels", *Journal of Biological Rhythms*, vol. 25, pp.208–16

Pillar Three: Nurture/Laugh More

Ghodsbin F *et al* (2015) "The effects of laughter therapy on general health of elderly people Referring to Jahandidegan Community Center in Shiraz, Iran, 2014: A randomized controlled trial", *International Journal of Community based Nursing and Midwifery*, vol. 3, pp.31–38

Pillar Three: Nurture/Change Your Response to Stress

Tsigos C and Chrousos G P (2002) "Hypothalamic-pituitary-adrenal axis, neuroendocrine factors and stress", *Journal of Psychosomatic Research*, vol. 53, pp.865–71

Pillar Three: Nurture/Be More Active

Ciloglu F *et al* (2005) "Exercise intensity and its effects on thyroid hormones", *Neuro Endocrinology Letters*, vol. 26, pp.830–34

Williams-Orlando C (2013) "Yoga therapy for anxiety: A case report", *Advances in Mind–Body Medicine*, vol. 27, pp.18–21

Pillar Three: Nurture/Nurture Your Thyroid

Zimmermann M B and Kohrle J (2002) "The impact of iron and selenium deficiencies on iodine and thyroid metabolism: biochemistry and relevance to public health", *Thyroid*, vol. 12, pp.867–78

Pillar Four: Cleanse/Cleanse your Body

Start your Day with a Cup of Warm Water and Lemon Juice

Fukuchi Y *et al* (2008) "Lemon polyphenols suppress diet-induced obesity by up-regulation of mRNA Levels of the enzymes involved in ß-oxidation in mouse white adipose tissue", *Journal of Clinical Biochemistry and Nutrition*, vol. 43, pp.201–09

Eat Some Ground Flaxseeds Every Day

Goyal A *et al* (2014) "Flax and flaxseed oil: an ancient medicine and modern functional food", *Journal of Food Science Technology*, vol. 51, pp.1633–53

Get Sweaty

Genuis S *et al* (2016) "Human elimination of organochlorine pesticides: blood, urine, and sweat study", *Biomed Research International*.

Genuis S J *et al* (2011) "Blood, urine, and sweat (BUS) study: Monitoring and elimination of bioaccumulated toxic elements", *Archives of Environmental Contamination and Toxicology*, vol. 61, pp.344–57

Genuis S *et al* (2012) "Human excretion of bisphenol A: Blood, urine, and sweat (BUS) study", *Journal of Environmental and Public Health*.

Pillar Four: Cleanse/Cleanse your Environment

Don't do Plastic

La Merrill M A (2016) "The economic legacy of endocrine disrupting chemicals", *The Lancet Diabetes and Endocrinology*, vol. 12, pp.961–62

Manage Your Cycle Ethically

Scranton A (2013) "Potential health effects of toxic chemicals in feminine care products", *Chem Fatale Report*. November 2013. *Women's Voices for the Earth*

Pillar Five: Move

Brooks K A and Carter J G (2013) "Overtraining, exercise and adrenal insufficiency", *Journal of Novel Physiotherapies*, vol. 3.

Warburton D E R et al (2006) "Health benefits of physical activity: the evidence", *Canadian Medical Association Journal*, vol. 174, pp.801–09

Pillar Six: Restore/Focus on Gratitude

Kini P *et al* (2016) "The effects of gratitude expression on neural activity", *NeuroImage*, vol. 128, pp.1–10

Wood A M *et al* (2008) "Gratitude uniquely predicts satisfaction with life: Incremental validity above the domains and facets of the five-factor model", *Personality and Individual Differences*, vol. 45, pp.49–54

Index

Cookery Notes

Standard level spoon measurements are used in all recipes.
1 tablespoon = one 15ml spoon
1 teaspoon = one 5ml spoon

Eggs should be organic, free-range medium unless otherwise stated. The Department of Health advises that eggs should not be consumed raw. This book contains dishes made with raw or lightly cooked eggs. It is prudent for more vulnerable people such as pregnant and nursing mothers, invalids, the elderly, babies and young children to avoid uncooked or lightly cooked dishes made with eggs. Once prepared these dishes should be kept refrigerated and used promptly.

Fresh herbs should be used unless otherwise stated. If unavailable use dried herbs as an alternative but halve the quantities stated.

Ovens should be preheated to the specific temperature – if using a fan-assisted oven, follow manufacturer's instructions for adjusting the time and the temperature.

Pepper should be freshly ground black pepper unless otherwise stated.

Salt should be sea salt unless otherwise stated.

This book includes dishes made with nuts and nut derivatives. It is advisable for those with known allergic reactions to nuts and nut derivatives and those who may be potentially vulnerable to these allergies, such as pregnant and nursing mothers, invalids, the elderly, babies and children, to avoid dishes made with nuts and nut oils. It is also prudent to check the labels of pre-prepared ingredients for the possible inclusion of nut derivatives.

Acknowledgements

I am so grateful for this opportunity to share my message and for all the people that have helped me achieve this. This book is a product of my knowledge and passion which has come to life through a lot of support from the incredible people in my life. Thank you to all those who provided support, bounced ideas, talked things over, read, wrote, offered comments, tested recipes, researched scientific papers and assisted in the editing, proofreading and design. Without you this would not have been possible.

A timeless thank you to my darling husband Ryan for his abundant love and for having supported, encouraged and believed in me, even when I haven't. Without you I would not be where I am today, you have helped me step outside my comfort zone and find my voice – I truly love you.

With a heart filled with love, I would like to thank our beautiful daughter Isabella Rose. You may have only just joined us, but the journey we took before we could finally meet you sculpted and nurtured my passion to find hormonal balance. Even before your birth, you taught me so much. I look forward to learning more from you.

I am delighted to thank my incredible family for their unwavering support through my studies to become a nutritional therapist, setting up my clinic and embarking on this journey of penning a book. A special mention for my inspiring mum Rosetta who has been my rock, my confidante and my biggest fan. It was her curiosity and knowledge of health and nutrition that inspired me to pursue this path. My beautiful sister Michela who has walked this path so closely with me, helped develop recipes with her incredible culinary flair and tested and tasted everything I have developed (except the fish dishes, still working on that!).

To my management company team at Crown Talent Group, Del Conboy, Sarah Walsh, Nicola Ibison, Deborah and Mark Hargreaves, Jonny Hurcombe and Amanda Preston from my literary agency, thank you for all you have done and continue to do.

Thank you to all at Octopus Publishing Group for giving me this opportunity and believing in my work – Stephanie Jackson and Polly Poulter, your patience and support has been incredible especially when I presented you with the biggest manuscript ever seen for editing, and also thank you for including my poop chart. Juliette Norsworthy and Lizzie Ballantyne your artistic excellence brought the book to life. Jen, Emily and Clare your food styling and photography make my recipes pop off the page, which will further inspire people to jump into the kitchen, and Ian thank you for spending the day with me and capturing me at my most relaxed.

To my tribe of strong women that support me every day and bring colour to my life. As the saying goes, 'behind every successful woman is a tribe of successful women who have her back'. I am blessed with such a tribe and I am so grateful for all of you. I would love to name you all but know that you are all in my heart.

To my mentors, colleagues and teachers, thank you for encouraging me and helping me expand my knowledge. To Mandy Lehto thank you for editing my proposal and helping me shape the message I wanted to share.

To my clients and followers, thank you for joining me on this journey – your embracement of my guidance gives me the strength to keep pushing, keep learning and spreading my message. I hope you will gain volumes from this book and find further balance.

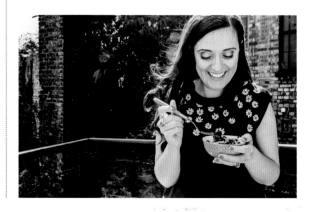